Atlas of Developmental Anomalies in Experimental Animals
実験動物発生異常アトラス

External Anomalies
外表異常

Edited by Project of the Terminology Committee of the Japanese Teratology Society

日本先天異常学会用語委員会　編集

FOREWORD

The first harmonized terminology (Version 1) of developmental anomalies in experimental animals, which was discussed by members of the International Federation of teratology Societies including North America, Europe and Japan, had been published in 1997 (Teratology, 55:249-292, 1997; Cong. Anom., 37:165-210,1997).   And then, the Japanese version of this terminology was made in the next year (Cong. Anom., 38:153-237, 1998).

The revised edition (Version 2) of this terminology had been published by the almost same members in 2009 (Cong. Anom., 49(3):123-246, 2009; Birth Defects Research (Part B), 86:227-327, 2009; Repro. Toxicol., 28:371-434, 2009). This version is described by simple words and is useful for laboratory technicians.

The Terminology committee of Japanese Teratology Society established "a Database of Congenital Anomalies in Laboratory animals" in the society homepage in 2010 and provided photographs of malformations and variations submitted by many companies in Japan until now. Submitted photographs were reviewed by a terminology project, some members in the committee, and were registered to the database mentioned above.

This textbook, "Atlas of Congenital Anomalies in Experimental Animals" gathered up photographs of external anomalies and their explanations. We will expect to be used by researches that conduct teratological studies and review the data of the reproductive and developmental toxicity.

はじめに

1960 年代のサリドマイド薬禍を契機として、化合物の暴露による先天異常発現が問題となり、多くの研究者により実験動物を用いた発生毒性研究が進められました。また、これら研究成果の科学的信憑性を担保するため、催奇形性試験や生殖発生毒性試験に関するガイドラインも各国の規制当局により制定・改訂され、今日に至っています。しかし、実験動物を用いた試験・研究においては、実際に観察する発生異常の診断は、臨床で用いられている先天異常用語を参考にして行っていたのが現状でした。1997 年に日欧米三極の研究者により実験動物での発生用語の統一が図られ、実験動物発生異常用語集 Version 1（Teratology, 55:249-292, 1997; Cong. Anom., 37:165-210,1997）が提示されました。また、翌年には日本語版として、「実験動物発生異常用語集」（Cong. Anom., 38:153-237, 1998）も発表されました。この用語集で用いられている所見名はいわゆる診断用語であり、試験・研究の実務担当者には扱いにくい面もあることから、より簡易な用語を用いた用語集 Version 2 として 2009 年に改訂されました（Cong. Anom., 49(3):123-246, 2009; Birth Defects Research (Part B), 86:227-327, 2009; Repro. Toxicol., 28:371-434, 2009）。

これを受けて、日本先天異常学会 用語委員会は2010年、学会ホームページに「実験動物先天異常データベース」を開設し、Version 2 に規定された用語集の日本語版を掲載すると共に、それらに該当する写真の公開を行っています。これまで多くの企業、施設のご協力により、貴重な異常・変異の写真を提供していただきました。この場を借り、お礼申し上げます。委員会では、審査プロジェクトを組み、メンバーにより写真及びその診断、説明の妥当性を審査し、上記データベースに登録してきました。

　本アトラスは、生殖発生毒性研究を実施される研究者や生殖発生毒性を評価される方々に活用いただける様、上記データベースを基に実験動物の外表異常の写真及びその説明をまとめたものです。

　また、近年、遺伝子解析技術の飛躍的な発展によって、先天異常学分野全般の研究が加速しています。今後、遺伝子改変動物の表現型の解析を通じた、遺伝子機能の決定、遺伝子変異とヒト遺伝性疾患の患者の症状の関係の研究の一層の展開が期待されます。遺伝子変異データがデジタルデータであるのに対して、表現型のデータはフォーマットの一定しないデータと見なされてきましたが、表現型をデジタル化可能なコードとして国際標準化しようとする動きが進んでいます。著者らはこの動きに呼応するかたちで、本アトラスに示される表現型に対してコードを示しました（Table 2 参照）。本アトラスが動物の胎児への薬物毒性の研究者のみならず、広く遺伝子改変動物やヒト遺伝性疾患の研究者にとって有用なレファレンスになればと願っています。

Smith CL et al. The Mammalian Phenotype Ontology as a tool for annotating, analyzing and comparing phenotypic information. Genome Biol. 6(1): R7, 2005

Kohler S et al. The Human Phenotype Ontology project: linking molecular biology and disease through phenotype data. Nucleic Acids Res. 42:D966, 2014.

協力企業・施設

アステラス製薬株式会社	株式会社ボゾリサーチセンター
塩野義製薬株式会社	小野薬品工業株式会社
株式会社新日本科学	大鵬薬品工業株式会社
第一三共株式会社	中外製薬株式会社
田辺三菱製薬株式会社	武田薬品工業株式会社
鳥取大学医学部	株式会社日本バイオリサーチセンター
財団法人食品農医薬品安全性評価センター	日産化学工業株式会社

Project members of the Terminology Committee in Japanese Teratology Society

Yojiro Ooshima

Michio Fujiwara (Astellas Pharma Inc.)

Kazuhiro Chihara (Sumitomo Dainippon Pharma Co., Ltd.)

Yuko Izumi (Takeda Pharmaceutical Company Ltd.)

Yoshihiro Katsumata (BoZo Research Center Inc.)

Hiroshi Sumida (Hiroshima International University)

Makoto Ema (AIST)

Kenjiro Kosaki (Keio University)

Advisors

Kohei Shiota (Shiga University of Medical Science)

Kok Wah Hew (Takeda Pharmaceutical Company Ltd., USA)

CONTENTS

Foreword

Table 1 List of External Anomalies 1

Table 2 Comparative List of This Atlas Findings, Mouse Phenotype, and Human Phenotype 20

Photographs of Normal Fetuses in Rats, Rabbits and Mice 23

Photographs of External Anomalies
   1. General 31
   2. Head and Neck 45
   3. Ear and Eye 57
   4. Face 69
   5. Limb 91
   6. Paw and Digit 101
   7. Tail 121
   8. Trunk 141

Table 1 List of External Anomalies

Region / Organ / Structure	Observation		Synonym or *Related Term*	Virsion 1 Code No.	Definition	Note	Photo
General 全身	Subcutaneous edema 皮下浮腫	Generalized 全身性	Anasarca 全身性浮腫	10001	An accumulation of interstitial fluid in subcutaneous connective tissue 皮下結合組織における間質液の全身性の貯溜		1-1
		Localized 局所性		10005	Localized accumulation of fluid 液体（間質液）の局所性の貯溜		
	Conjoined twins 二重体		*Omphalosite* 臍帯寄生体 臍帯栄養児	10002	Monozygotic twins with variable incomplete separation into two during cleavage or early stages of embryogenesis 卵割あるいは胚発生の早い時期に種々の程度で不完全に2つに分かれた一卵性双生児	Site and extent of fusion should be described. 癒合の部位および範囲を記述する。	1-2
	Distended abdomen 腹部膨満			New	Abdomen appears larger than normal. 腹部が正常より大きく見える。	May be due to presence of fluid in abdomen or enlarged organs. 腹部の液体貯留あるいは腫大した器官による場合がある。	
	Fetus or pup/neonate 胎児、出生児/新生児	Discolored 変色	Skin discolored 皮膚変色	New	Generalized or localized region of abnormal color (other than pale) 全身あるいは局所領域の異常色（蒼白以外）	See also "General – Fetus or pup/neonate Pale" 「全身－胎児、出生児/新生児の蒼白」を参照	
		Large 大型(化)		New		Relative to normal 正常と比較	
		Pale 蒼白		New	Generalized absence of color when compared to a normal specimen 正常例と比較した場合の色の全身性欠如	See also "General – Fetus or pup/neonate Discolored" 「全身－胎児、出生児/新生児の変色」を参照	
		Small 小型(化)	Runt 矮小	New		Relative to normal 正常と比較	
	Subcutaneous hemorrhage 皮下出血		Petechia, Purpura, Ecchymosis, Hematoma 点状出血、紫斑、斑状出血、血腫	10004	An accumulation of extravasated blood beneath the skin 皮下における溢血の貯溜		1-3

Table 1 List of External Anomalies

Region / Organ / Structure	Observation	Synonym or *Related Term*	Virsion 1 Code No.	Definition	Note	Photo
	Skin 皮膚	Absent 欠損	Cutis aplasia 皮膚無形成	10003	Localized region of no skin development 局所的に皮膚の発生がないこと	EC (Editor comment): Occasionally general region 編者注：全身性の場合もある。	1-4
		Discolored 変色		New	Localized region of abnormal color 局所領域の異常色	See also "General-Fetus or pup/neonate discolored" 「全身―胎児、出生児/新生児の変色」を参照	
		Lesion 病変	Cutis lesion 皮膚病変	New	Localized region of abnormal skin 局所的な皮膚の異常		
		Tag 付属物		New	Small appendage of skin 皮膚の小さな付着物	EC: The tag at digits is pendulous digit (New). See Photo 6-7 編者注：指趾における付着物は浮遊指・趾(New)とする。	1-5
Head / Neck 頭部/頸部	Acephalostomia 無頭有口			10008	Absence of head but with the presence of mouth-like orifice in the neck region 頭部が欠損しているが、口様の孔が頸部にあるもの	EC: Acrania is a term for skeletal findings. 編者注：無頭蓋(Acrania)は骨格用語	2-1
	Anencephaly 無脳			10010	Absence of the cranial region of the head, with the brain absent or reduced 脳の欠損あるいは減形成を伴った頭蓋部位の欠損	EC: Acrania is a term for skeletal findings. 編者注：無頭蓋(Acrania)は骨格用語	
	Cranial meningocele 頭蓋髄膜瘤			10016	Herniation of meninges through a defect in skull 頭蓋骨欠損による髄膜のヘルニア	EC: Note to confuse with meningo-encephalocele (10017) and meningohydro-encephalocele (New). See Photos 2-7 and 2-8. 編者注：髄膜脳瘤(10017)や髄膜水脳瘤(New)との比較に注意	2-6
	Cranioschisis 頭蓋裂			10011	Fissure of the cranial region of the head with varying degrees of the brain exposed 様々な程度の脳の露出を伴う頭蓋部位の裂	EC: Note to confuse with holorachischisis (10110). 編者注：脊椎にも及ぶ場合は完全脊椎裂(10110)	2-2

Table 1 List of External Anomalies

Region / Organ / Structure	Observation		Synonym or *Related Term*	Virsion 1 Code No.	Definition	Note	Photo
	Exencephaly 外脳			10013	Brain protrudes outside the skull due to absence of all or part of the cranial vault. 頭蓋の全てあるいは一部の欠損のために脳が頭骨から外に突出している「編者注：脳室壁の露出(脳の反転)を伴う」。	Erosion of brain tissue has not occurred as in Anencephaly 無脳(症)でみられるような脳組織のびらんはみられない。	2-3
	External aural fistula 外耳瘻孔			New	An opening to a cyst produced by a persistent lateral cervical sinus or reduplicated 1st pharyngeal cleft usually located ventral to the ear. 通常，耳の腹側に開口する嚢で，(側部の)頸洞の残存あるいは第1咽頭溝(鰓溝)の重複により発生する。		
	Head 頭部	Absent 欠損	Acephaly 無頭(症)	10009	Absence of the head 頭部の欠損		2-4
		Domed ドーム状		10012	Cranial region of head appears more elevated and rounded than normal. 頭蓋が正常より高く丸くなっている。	May or may not be associated with hydrocephaly. 水頭(症)を伴う場合と伴わない場合がある。	2-5
		Large 大型(化)	Macrocephaly 大頭(症)	10015	Disproportionately large head 体躯に比して頭部が不釣合いに大きい。		
		Misshapen 形態異常		New			
		Small 小型(化)	Leptocephaly, Microcephaly, Nanocephaly 狭小(化)頭蓋(症)、小頭症	10018	Disproportionately small head 体躯に比して頭部が不釣合いに小さい。		
	Iniencephaly 後頭孔脳脱出			10014	Exposure of occipital brain and upper spinal cord tissue; involves extreme retroflection of the head 後頭部の脳および上部脊髄組織の露出；頭部の極端な後屈を伴う。		

Table 1   List of External Anomalies

Region / Organ / Structure	Observation		Synonym or *Related Term*	Virsion 1 Code No.	Definition	Note	Photo
	Meningo-encephalocele 髄膜脳瘤		Encephalo-meningocele 脳髄膜ヘルニア	10017	Herniation of brain and meninges through a cranial opening 頭蓋の開口による脳および髄膜のヘルニア	May or may not be covered by skin. EC: Note to confuse with cranial meningocele (10016) and meningohydro-encephalocele (New). See Photos 2-6 and 2-8. This may be "Encephalocele" concluding meningohydro-encephalocele. 皮膚で被われている場合といない場合がある。編者注：頭蓋髄膜瘤(10016)や髄膜水脳瘤(New)との比較に注意。髄膜水脳瘤を含めて脳瘤と総称する場合がある。	2-7
	Meningohydro-encephalocele 髄膜水脳瘤			New	Herniation of brain, cerebral ventricle, and meninges through a defect in skull 頭蓋欠損による脳、脳室および髄膜のヘルニア	EC: Note to confuse with cranial meningocele (10016) and meningoencephalocele (10017). See Photos 2-6 and 2-7. This may be "Encephalocele" concluding meningo-encephalocele. 編者注：頭蓋髄膜瘤(10016)や髄膜脳瘤(10017)との比較に注意。脳髄膜瘤を含めて脳瘤と総称する場合がある。	2-8
	Narrow head 狭頭		*Craniostenosis* 狭頭(症)	New			
Ear 耳	Pinna 耳介	Absent 欠損	Anotia 無耳(症)	10019	Absence of external ear 外耳の欠損		
		Fused 癒合	Synotia 合耳(症)	10024	Fusion or abnormal approximation of pinnae below the face 顔より下位での耳介の癒合あるいは異常な接近		
		Large 大型(化)	Long pinna,Macrotia 大耳介、巨耳(症)	10020	Disproportionately large external ear 体躯に比して外耳が不釣合いに大きい。		

Table 1   List of External Anomalies

Region / Organ / Structure	Observation		Synonym or *Related Term*	Virsion 1 Code No.	Definition	Note	Photo
		Malpositioned 位置異常	Low set pinna 耳介低位	10021			3-1
		Misshapen 形態異常		10023			
		Small 小型(化)	Microtia, Short pinna 小耳介、小耳(症)	10022	Disproportionately small external ear 体躯に比して外耳が不釣合いに小さい。		3-2
Eye 眼	Cryptophthalmia 潜在眼球		Cryptophthalmos 潜在眼球	10026	Skin continuous over eye(s) without formation of eyelid(s) 眼瞼の形成がなく、皮膚が眼球全体を被っている。	May be associated with micro- or anophthalmia 小眼球あるいは無眼球を伴っている場合がある。	
	Cyclopia 単眼		Monophthalmia, Single eyeball, Synophthalmia 一眼奇形、単眼球、合眼(症)	10027	Single median orbit; eyeball(s) can be absent, completely or incompletely fused 中央に位置する一つの眼窩；眼球は欠損しているか、完全あるいは不完全に癒合している。	Snout may be absent or appear as a frontonasal appendage (proboscis) above the orbit 鼻が欠損している場合と、眼窩の上に前頭鼻部の付属物(象鼻)としてみえる場合がある。	3-3
	Eye 眼	Malpositioned 位置異常		10030			
		Open 開存		10033	Eyeball visible 眼球がみえる。	EC: May be "Ablepharia: absence of eyelid" or "Open eyelid" concluding eyelid fissure (10034). See Photo 3-7. 編者注：眼瞼の欠損(無眼瞼症)による場合があり、また、眼瞼裂(10034)を含めて眼瞼開裂(Open eyelid)と総称する場合がある。	3-4
		Protruding 突出	Exophthalmos Exophthalmia, Proptosis, 眼球突出	10029	Excessive protrusion of the eyeball 眼球の過度の突出		3-5

Table 1　　List of External Anomalies

Region / Organ / Structure	Observation		Synonym or *Related Term*	Virsion 1 Code No.	Definition	Note	Photo
	Eye bulge 眼部隆起	Absent 欠損		10025		Check for abnormalities of eye prior to opening of the eyelid May be associated with micro- or anophthalmia 眼瞼が開く前に眼の異常を調べる。小眼球あるいは無眼球を伴っている場合がある。	
		Large 大型(化)		10028		May be associated with macrophthalmia. 巨眼球を伴っている場合がある。	
		Small 扁平(化)		10035		May be associated with microphthalmia. 小眼球を伴っている場合がある。	**3-6**
	Eyelid 眼瞼	Fissure 裂	Palpebral coloboma 眼瞼コロボーマ	10034	A notch or fissure of the eyelid 眼瞼の切痕あるいは裂	EC: May be "Ablepharia: absence of eyelid" or "Open eyelid" concluding open eye (10033). See Photo 3-4. 編者注：眼瞼の欠損(無眼瞼症)による場合があり、また、眼開存(10033)を含めて眼瞼開裂(Open eyelid)と総称する場合がある。	**3-7**
		Short 短小	Microblepharia 小眼瞼(症)	10031	Short vertical dimension of eyelid 眼瞼の縦幅の短小		
Face 顔面	Face 顔面	Cleft 裂	Prosoposchisis 顔面裂	10036	Fissure of the face. 顔面の裂	EC: May be "Aprosopia" when it is severe hypogenesis of the face. Note to confuse with cleft upper jaw (New) and cranioschisis (10011). See Photos 2-2 and 4-5. 編者注：顔面の形成不全が著しい場合、無顔症と総称する場合がある。上顎裂(New)や頭蓋裂(10011)と区分に注意。	**4-1**

Table 1 List of External Anomalies

Region / Organ / Structure	Observation		Synonym or *Related Term*	Virsion 1 Code No.	Definition	Note	Photo
	Jaw, lower (Mandible) 下顎	Absent 欠損	Agnathia 無顎(症)	10047			4-2
		Cleft 裂	Gnathoschisis, Split mandible 顎裂, 下顎裂	10056			4-3
		Large 大型(化)	Mandibular macrognathia, *Long lower jaw Protruding lower jaw, Prognathia* 巨下顎、下顎突出, 顎前突出(症)	10057			
		Small 小型(化)	Brachygnathia, Micromandible, *Short lower jaw* 小顎(症), 小下顎、下顎短小	10058			4-4
	Jaw, upper (Maxilla) 上顎	Cleft 裂	Gnathoschisis, Split maxilla 顎裂, 上顎裂	New		EC: Note to confuse with cleft face (10036). See Photo 4-1. 編者注：程度の差で、顔面裂(10036)と区分。	4-5
		Large 大型(化)	Maxillary macrognathia, *Long lower jaw Protruding upper jaw, Prognathia* 巨上顎, 上顎突出, 顎前突出(症)	10059			
		Small 小型(化)	Maxillary micrognathia, Micromaxilla, *Short upper jaw* 小顎(症), 小上顎、上顎短小	10060			4-6
	Lip 唇	Cleft 裂	Cheiloschisis 唇裂	10051	Fissure of the upper lip 上唇に裂が生じている。		4-7
	Mouth 口	Absent 欠損	Astomia 無口(症)	10050			4-8

Table 1　　List of External Anomalies

Region / Organ / Structure	Observation		Synonym or *Related Term*	Virsion 1 Code No.	Definition	Note	Photo
		Large 大型(化)	Macrostomia, *Wide mouth* 巨口，広口	10055			**4-9**
		Misshapen 形態異常		New			
		Small 小型(化)	Microstomia 小口(症)	10062			
	Naris 鼻孔	Absent 欠損	*Atretic* 閉鎖	10042			
		Fused 癒合		New			
		Malpositioned 位置異常		10039			
		Single 単	Mononaris 単鼻孔	10044			
		Small 狭小(化)		New			
	Palate 口蓋	Cleft 裂	Palatoschisis, Uranoschisis 口蓋裂	10052	Fissure of the palate 口蓋に裂が生じている。		**4-10**
		High-arched 高アーチ状	編者注：高口蓋	10053	Roof of mouth higher than normal 口腔の天井部が通常より高い。		
	Palatal rugae 口蓋ヒダ	Absent 欠損		New	Absence of one or more rugae 1つ以上のヒダの欠損		
		Interrupted 離断		New			
		Misaligned 不整列	Asymmetrically aligned palatal rugae, *Irregular palatal rugae* 非対称性口蓋ヒダ，不規則性口蓋ヒダ	10063			**4-11**

Table 1   List of External Anomalies

Region / Organ / Structure	Observation		Synonym or *Related Term*	Virsion 1 Code No.	Definition	Note	Photo
		Misshapen 形態異常	*Bifurcated palatal rugae, Discontinuous palatal rugae, Short palatal rugae* 分岐状口蓋ヒダ, 不連続性口蓋ヒダ, 短口蓋ヒダ	10064			4-12
		Supernumerary 過剰		New			
	Papillae 乳頭	Absent 欠損		New	Dermal projections, generally associated with whiskers 皮膚の突起物であり，通常はヒゲを伴っている。		
		Fused 癒合		New			
		Malpositioned 位置異常		New			
	Proboscis 象鼻			10043	Tubular projection replaces the snout 鼻の代わりに筒状の突出がある。		4-13
	Snout 鼻	Absent 欠損	Arhinia 無鼻	10038			
		Large 大型(化)	*Long* 長鼻	New			
		Malpositioned 位置異常		10040			
		Misshapen 形態異常		10041			4-14
		Small 小型(化)	*Short* 短鼻	10045			
	Tongue 舌	Absent 欠損	Aglossia 無舌	10046			

Table 1   List of External Anomalies

Region / Organ / Structure	Observation	Synonym or *Related Term*	Virsion 1 Code No.	Definition	Note	Photo
		Altered surface texture 表面組織変化		New		May be generalized or localized; location and description should be provided. 全体あるいは局所の場合がある；位置と特徴を記述する。	
		Large 大型(化)	Macroglossia, *Long tongue* 巨舌, *長舌*	10054		May be protruding 口外に突出している場合がある。	
		Misshapen 形態異常		New			
		Protruding 突出		10065			**4-15**
		Small 小型(化)	Microglossia, *Short tongue* 小舌(症), *短舌*	10061			
		Split 裂		New			
	Tongue, frenulum 舌、小帯	Fused to floor of mouth 口腔底部癒合	Ankyloglossia 舌強直	10048	Shortness or absence of the frenulum of the tongue; tongue fused to the floor of the mouth 舌小帯の短小あるいは欠損；舌が口腔底部と癒合している。		**4-16**
	Tooth 歯	Absent 欠損	Anodontia, Edentia 無歯(症)	10049	Absence of one or more teeth 1本以上の歯の欠損		
		Asymmetric 非対称		New			
		Bent 弯曲		New			
		Discolored 変色		New			
		Erupted 萌出		New			
		Fused 癒合		New			
		Large 大型(化)		New			

Table 1   List of External Anomalies

Region / Organ / Structure	Observation		Synonym or *Related Term*	Virsion 1 Code No.	Definition	Note	Photo
		Malpositioned 位置異常		New			
		Not erupted 無萌出		New			
		Small 小型(化)		New			
	Whiskers ヒゲ	Absent 欠損		New			
Limb (fore- or hind-) 肢(前肢、後肢)	Hemimelia 半肢			10068	Absence or shortening of the distal two segments of limb 肢の先端2分節(前腕と手あるいは下腿と足)の欠損あるいは短小	May be further characterized, at skeletal examination, as being fibular, radial, tibial, or ulnar 橈骨、尺骨、脛骨、腓骨を骨格検査でさらに特定する場合がある。	
	Limb 肢	Absent 欠損	Amelia, Ectromelia 無肢(症)、欠肢(症)	10066	Complete absence of one or more limbs 一本以上の肢の完全な欠損	Fleshy tab may be present 肉様付属物が存在している場合がある。	5-1
		Bent 弯曲	Bowed limb, Curved limb 弯曲肢	10067			
		Fused 癒合	*Symmelia* 合肢(症)	10075			
		Hyperextension 過伸展		10069	The excessive extension or straightening of a limb or a joint. 肢あるいは関節の過度の伸展	Limb cannot be flexed Joint can be specified. See also 10086 肢を曲げられない 関節を特定する。 10086を参照	5-2
		Hyperflexion 過屈曲	Flexed limb 屈曲肢	10070	The excessive flexion or bending of a limb or a joint. 肢あるいは関節の過度の屈曲または弯曲	Limb cannot be straightened. Joint can be specified. See also 10087 肢を伸展できない 関節を特定する。 10087を参照	
		Large 大型(化)	Macromelia, *Long limb* 巨肢(症)	10071			

Table 1 List of External Anomalies

Region / Organ / Structure	Observation		Synonym or *Related Term*	Virsion 1 Code No.	Definition	Note	Photo
		Malrotated 異常回転		10072	Limb turned toward the center (i.e., inward rotation) or the periphery (i.e., outward rotation) 肢が中心(内側回転)あるいは外側(外側回転)に向かっている。		**5-3**
		Small 小型(化)	*Brachymelia,* Micromelia, Nanomelia, *Short limb* 短肢, 小肢(症), 矮肢(症)	10073			**5-4**
	Phocomelia フォコメリア		Ectromelia 欠肢(症)	10074	Reduction or absence of proximal portion of limb, with the paws being attached to the trunk of the body 肢の基部の減形成あるいは欠損、手足首が体躯に付いている。		**5-5**
Paw / Digit (fore- or hind-) 手足/指趾 (前、後)	Digit 指趾	Absent 欠損	Adactyly 無指(趾)(症)	10077	Absence of all digits 全指〈趾〉の欠損	See Digit, few (Ectrodactyly) for absence of some but not all digits. 全指<趾>ではなく、一部の指<趾>の欠損については、「Digit, few 少指<趾> (乏指<趾>)」を参照	**6-1**
		Few 少ない	Ectrodactyly, Oligodactyly 欠指(趾) (症), 乏指(趾) (症)	10080	Absence of one or more, but not all, digit(s) 全部ではないが、1本以上の指〈趾〉の欠損	Expected skeletal alterations include absence of all phalanges in each affected digit 影響を受けたそれぞれの指〈趾〉で、全ての指〈趾〉骨の欠損を含む骨の変化が予想される。	**6-2**

Table 1   List of External Anomalies

Region / Organ / Structure	Observation	Synonym or *Related Term*	Virsion 1 Code No.	Definition	Note	Photo
	Fused 癒合	Ankylodactyly, Syndactyly, Webbed digits 強直指(趾)(症), 合指(趾)(症), 水かき状指(趾)	10091	Partial or complete fusion of, or webbing between, digits 指〈趾〉の部分的あるいは完全な癒合、あるいは指間が水かき状になっている。	Includes bony, cartilaginous, and/or soft tissue EC: May be "Polysyndactyly" when this is supernumerary digit (10088). 骨、軟骨および/あるいは軟組織を含む。 編者注：多指(趾)を伴うものを多合指(趾)とする場合がある。	6-3
	Large 大型(化)	Dactylomegaly, Macrodactyly 巨指(趾)	10081			6-4
	Malpositioned 位置異常	Clinodactyly, Camptodactyly 斜指(趾)(症)、屈指(趾)(症)	10083	Deflection of digit(s) from the central axis 中心軸からの指〈趾〉のゆがみ(それること)	Includes fixed flexion deformity of digit(s). Confirmed by skeletal examination to exclude the possibility of artifact. 指の固定屈曲変形を含むアーチファクトの可能性を除くために、骨格検査によって確かめる。	6-5
	Misshapen 形態異常		10085			6-6
	Pendulous 有茎性	浮遊指(趾)	New	Digit attached by a thread of tissue. 索状組織でつながっている。		6-7
	Small 小型(化)	*Brachydactyly*, Microdactyly, *Short digit* 短指、小指(趾)(症)	10079		Expected skeletal alterations include absence or shortening of phalanx(ges) 指<趾>骨の欠損あるいは短小を含む骨の変化が予想される。	6-8

Table 1   List of External Anomalies

Region / Organ / Structure	Observation		Synonym or *Related Term*	Virsion 1 Code No.	Definition	Note	Photo
		Supernumerary 過剰	Polydactyly 多指(趾)(症)	10088		Can be pendulous. EC: May be "Polysyndactyly" when this is fused digit (10091). 有茎性のことがある。 編者注：合指(趾)を伴うものを多合指(趾)とする場合がある。	6-9
	Claw 爪	Absent 欠損		10076		Refers to distal-most tip, nail 指趾の最末端や爪(nail)にも用いられる。	6-10
		Malpositioned 位置異常		10082		Refers to distal-most tip, nail 指趾の最末端や爪(nail)にも用いられる。	
		Small 小型(化)		10089		Refers to distal-most tip, nail 指趾の最末端や爪(nail)にも用いられる。	6-11
	Paw 手<足>	Absent 欠損	Acheiria, Acheiropodia, Apodia 無手(症)、無手無足(症)、無足(症)	10078			
		Fused 癒合	Sympodia 合足	10092		Refers to hind paws in bipeds. 二足動物では後足に用いられる。	
		Malrotated 異常回転	編者注：日本では 内反手(足)、外反手(足)の使用が許容される	10084	Paw turned toward the center (i.e., inward) or the periphery (i.e., outward) 手足首から先が中心(内側)あるいは外側に向いている。		6-12
		Hyperextension 過伸展		10086	The excessive extension or straightening of a paw. 手足首から先の過度の伸展	Carpus or tarsus cannot be flexed. 手根または足根を曲げられない。	
		Hyperflexion 過屈曲	Flexed paw, Tarsal flexure, Carpal flexure 屈曲手(足)	10087	The excessive flexion or bending of a paw. 手足首から先の過度の屈曲あるいは弯曲	Carpus or tarsus cannot be straightened. 手根または足根を伸展できない。	6-13

Table 1   List of External Anomalies

Region / Organ / Structure	Observation		Synonym or *Related Term*	Virsion 1 Code No.	Definition	Note	Photo
		Small 小型	Microcheiria 小手(症)	10090			
Tail 尾	Tail 尾	Absent 欠損	Acaudia, Anury 無尾	10093			7-1
		Bent 屈曲	Angulated tail 屈曲尾	10094	Shaped like an angle 折れ曲がっている。		7-2
		Bifurcated 二又	Branched tail, Double-tipped tail, Forked tail 分岐尾，二又尾，フォーク状尾	10097	Tail divided or split 分裂あるいは分岐した尾		7-3
		Blunt-tipped 鈍端		10095	Rounded or flat at the end, not tapered 先端が丸いか平らで、先細ではない。		
		Curled 巻いた	Curly tail 巻尾	10096	Curved into nearly a full circle, or coiled ほぼ一巻きしているあるいはコイル状となっている。		7-4
		Discolored 変色		New	Generalized or localized discoloration of tail 尾の全部あるいは部分的な変色		
		Fleshy tab 肉様付属物		10098	Small tag of tissue at tip of tail. 尾の先端部での小さな付属物状の組織		7-5
		Hooked カギ状		10099	Approximately 180 degree bend or curve of the tail 尾が約180°折れ曲がっているか、弯曲している。		7-6
		Kinked 曲		10100	Localized undulation(s) of the tail 尾が局部的に波打っている。		7-7
		Long 長い		New			
		Malpositioned 位置異常		10101			
		Misshapen 形態異常		New			7-8

Table 1   List of External Anomalies

Region / Organ / Structure	Observation		Synonym or *Related Term*	Virsion 1 Code No.	Definition	Note	Photo
		Narrow 狭窄	Constricted tail 狭窄尾	10102		Should be specified as entire length or localized. 全体か局所かを区別(記載)する。	7-9
		Small 小型(化)	*Brachyury, Short tail* 短尾	10103			7-10
		Thread-like 索状	Filamentous tail, Filiform tail 糸状尾	10104		Should be specified as entire length or localized. 全体か局所かを区別(記載)する。	7-11
Trunk 躯幹	Anus 肛門	Absent 欠損	Anal atresia, Aproctia, Imperforate anus, Non-patent anus 鎖肛, 無肛門 (症), 肛門閉鎖	10105	Absence or closure of the anal opening 肛門の欠損あるいは閉鎖	May be associated with absent/threadlike tail. 尾の欠損/索状尾を伴っている場合がある。	8-1
		Large 大型(化)		New		編者注：大腸脱出参照	
		Small 小型(化)		10118			8-2
	Anogenital distance (AGD) 肛門生殖突起間距離	Decreased 短縮		10107	Shortened distance between anus and genital tubercle 肛門と生殖突起の間の距離(AGD)の短縮		
		Increased 延長		10112	Increased distance between anus and genital tubercle 肛門と生殖突起の間の距離(AGD)の延長		
	Externalized heart 心臓逸所		Ectopia cordis 逸脱心	10108	Heart displaced outside thoracic cavity 胸腔外への心臓の逸脱		8-3

Table 1   List of External Anomalies

Region / Organ / Structure	Observation		Synonym or *Related Term*	Virsion 1 Code No.	Definition	Note	Photo
	Gastroschisis 腹壁裂		Laparoschisis, Schistocelia 腹裂奇形	10109	Fissure of abdominal wall, not involving the umbilicus, and usually accompanied by protrusion of viscera which may or may not be covered by a membranous sac 臍の部分以外での腹壁の裂で、通常、器官の突出を伴う(膜性の嚢に被われている場合と被われていない場合がある)。	May be further defined as medial (gastroschisis) or lateral fissure (laparoschisis) 正中の(gastroschisis)あるいは側面の裂け目(laparoschisis)として細分類する場合がある。	8-4
	Genital tubercle 生殖突起	Absent 欠損		10106			8-5
		Large 大型(化)		New			
		Misshapen 形態異常		New			
		Small 小型(化)		10119			
	Holorachischisis 完全脊椎裂		EC: Cranioraschisis 編者注：頭蓋脊椎破裂	10110	Fissure of the entire spinal column 脊柱管全体の裂		8-6
	Hypospadias 尿道下裂			10111	Urethra opening on the underside of the penis or on the perineum 陰茎の下面あるいは会陰に尿道が開口している。	Not readily apparent in fetuses or soon after birth 胎児あるいは出生直後の児では明瞭でない。	8-7
	Kyphosis 脊柱後弯			10113	Increased dorsal convexity in the curvature of the spinal column as viewed from the side 側方から見たとき、脊柱が背側方向へ凸弯曲している。		
	Large intestine 大腸	Prolapsed 脱出		New	Protrusion of large intestine through anus 肛門からの大腸の脱出	May be associated with large anus 肛門大型化を伴っている場合がある。	
	Lordosis 脊柱前弯			10114	Increased dorsal concavity in the curvature of the spinal column as viewed from the side 側方から見たとき、脊柱が背側方向へ凹弯曲している。		

Table 1　List of External Anomalies

Region / Organ / Structure	Observation	Synonym or *Related Term*	Virsion 1 Code No.	Definition	Note	Photo
	Omphalocele 臍帯ヘルニア	Exomphalos, 臍突出	10115	A defect in the abdominal wall at the umbilicus, through which the intestines and other viscera protrude. These may or may not be covered by a thin, translucent sac composed of peritoneum and amnion. 腸および他の内臓器官が突出する臍部分の腹壁の欠損。これらは、腹膜と羊膜の薄い半透明の嚢によって覆われている場合といない場合がある。		**8-11**
	Pelvic region 骨盤部	Narrow 狭窄		New	Hindlimbs located more medially than normal 後肢が通常よりも内側に位置する。		
	Scoliosis 脊柱側弯		10116	Lateral curvature of the spinal column 脊柱が側方へ弯曲している。		
	Spina bifida 二分脊椎	Spinal meningocele, Spinal meningomyelocele, Spinal myelocele, Spinal myelomeningocele, Rachischisis EC: Myeloschisis 髄膜瘤，髄膜脊髄瘤，脊髄瘤，脊髄髄膜瘤，脊椎(破)裂	10120	A family of defects in the closure of the spinal column 一連の脊柱管閉鎖障害	May be covered with skin (spina bifida occulta) or not covered with skin (spina bifida aperta); may involve protrusion of spinal cord and/or meninges. 皮膚に覆われている場合（潜在性二分脊椎）と覆われていない（開放性二分脊椎）場合がある；脊髄または髄膜の突出を伴っている場合がある。	**8-8**
	Thoracogastroschisis 胸腹壁裂	Thoracoceloschisis 胸腹壁裂(症)	10121	Fissure of thoracic and abdominal walls with thoracic and abdominal viscera, or major parts thereof, exposed ventrally 胸腹壁の裂で胸腔および腹腔内器官あるいはそれら大部分の腹側からの逸脱を伴う。		**8-9**

Table 1 List of External Anomalies

Region / Organ / Structure	Observation	Synonym or *Related Term*	Virsion 1 Code No.	Definition	Note	Photo
	Thoracoschisis 胸壁裂			10122	Fissure of thoracic wall 胸壁の裂	Thoracic viscera may be herniated 胸部器官のヘルニアの場合がある。	
	Thorax 胸郭	Narrow 狭窄	Thoracostenosis 胸郭狭窄	10123	Narrowness of the thoracic region 胸郭の狭窄		
	Trunk 躯幹	Large 大型(化)	*Long trunk*	New			
		Small 小型(化)	*Short trunk 短躯*	10117			**8-10**
	Umbilicus 臍	Hernia ヘルニア		10124	Protrusion of a skin-covered segment of the gastrointestinal tract and/or greater omentum through a defect in the abdominal wall at the umbilicus, the herniated mass being circumscribed and covered with skin; or protrusion of skin-covered viscera through the umbilical ring with prominence of the navel 胃腸管ないし大網が臍部の腹壁の欠陥部から突出している状態。脱出した臓器塊は境界明瞭で皮膚に覆われている；あるいは臍輪から内臓が突出し、臍が隆起している状態。		**8-12**
		Malpositioned 位置異常		New			

Table 2 Comparative List of This Atlas Findings, Mouse Phenotype, and Human Phenotype

Photo No.	Atlas Term	MP No.	MP Term	HP No.	HP Term
1-1	Anasarca 全身性皮下浮腫	0011738	Anasarca	0012050	Anasarca
1-3	Subcutaneous hemorrhage 皮下出血	0011514	Skin hemorrhage	0001933	Subcutaneous hemorrhage
1-4	Absent skin 皮膚欠損	0003941	Abnormal skin development	0001057	Aplasia cutis congenita
1-5	Skin tag 皮膚付属物	0009931	Abnormal skin appearance	0010609	Skin tags
2-2	Cranioschisis 頭蓋裂	0000919	Cranioschisis		
2-3	Exencephaly 外脳	0000914	Exencephaly		
2-4	Absent head 頭部欠損	0009579	Acephaly		
2-5	Domed head ドーム状頭部	0000440	Domed cranium		
2-6	Cranial meningocele 頭蓋髄膜瘤	0012259	Meningocele	0002435	Meningocele
2-7	Meningo-encephalocele 髄膜脳瘤	0012260	Encephalomeningocele	0002084	Encephalocele
3-1	Malpositioned pinna 耳介位置異常	0000023	Abnormal ear distance/position	0000357	Abnormal location of ears
3-2	Small pinna 耳介小型(化)	0000018	Small ears	0008551	Microtia
3-3	Cyclopia 単眼	0005163	Cyclopia	0009914	Cyclopia
3-4	Open eye 眼開存	0001302	Eyelid open at birth		
3-5	Protruding eye 眼突出	0002750	Exophthalmos	0000520	Proptosis
4-1	Cleft face 顔面裂	0008797	Facial cleft	0002006	Facial cleft
4-2	Absent lower jaw 無顎	0000087	Absent mandible	0009939	Mandibular aplasia
4-3	Split/cleft mandible 下顎裂	0000114	Cleft chin	0010752	Cleft mandible
4-4	Small mandible 下顎小型化	0002639 0004592	Micrognathia Small mandible	0000347	Micrognathia
4-5	Cleft maxilla 上顎裂	0000455	Abnormal maxilla morphology	0000326	Abnormality of the maxilla
4-6	Cleft lip 唇裂	0005170	Cleft lip	0000204	Cleft upper lip
4-7	Absent mouth 無口	0000453	Absent mouth	0000153	Abnormality of the mouth
4-8	Large mouth 巨口	0009881	Macrostomia	0000154	Wide mouth
4-9	Cleft palate 口蓋裂	0000111	Cleft palate	0000175	Cleft palate
4-10	Misaligned palatal rugae 口蓋ヒダ不整列	0009652	Abnormal palatal rugae morphology	0000174	Abnormality of the palate
4-11	Mishapen palatal rugae 口蓋ヒダ形態異常	0009652	Abnormal palatal rugae morphology	0000174	Abnormality of the palate
4-12	Proboscis 象鼻	0006290	Proboscis	0012806	Proboscis
4-13	Misshapen snout 鼻形態異常	0002233	Abnormal nose morphology	0005105	Abnormal nasal morphology
4-14	Protruding tongue 舌突出	0009908	Protruding tongue	0010808	Protruding tongue
4-15	Ankyloglossia 舌癒合	0013264	Tongue ankylosis	0010296	Ankyloglossia
4-16	Small upper jaw (maxilla) 上顎小型化	0004540	Small maxilla	0000327	Hypoplasia of the maxilla
5-1	Absent limb 肢欠損	0000549	Absent limbs	0009827	Amelia
5-2	Hyperextension of limb 過伸展肢	0002109	Abnormal limb morphology	0005750	Contractures of the joints of the lower limbs
5-3	Malrotated limb 異常回転肢	0002109	Abnormal limb morphology		
5-4	Micromelia 小肢	0008736	Micromelia	0002983	Micromelia
5-5	Phocomelia フォコメリア	0002109	Abnormal limb morphology	0009829	Phocomelia

MP: Mouse phenotype
HP: Human phenotype
In some cases, MP and HP terms indicate a more general description for the Atlas term.

Table 2 Comparative List of This Atlas Findings, Mouse Phenotype, and Human Phenotype

Photo No.	Atlas Term	MP No.	MP Term	HP No.	HP Term
6-1	Absent digit　無趾	0000561	Adactyly	0009776	Adactyly
6-2	Few digit　欠指趾	0005230	Ectrodactyly	0100257	Ectrodactyly
6-3	Fused digit　合指趾	0000564	Syndactyly	0001159	Syndactyly
6-4	Large digit　巨大指趾	0013149	Macrodactyly	0004099	Macrodactyly
6-5	Malpositioned digit　指趾位置異常	0006253	Clinodactyly	0030084	Clinodactyly
		0003807	Camptodactyly	0012385	Camptodactyly
6-6	Misshapen digit　指趾形態異常	0002110	Abnormal digit morphology	0001171	Split hand
6-8	Small digit　短指趾	0002544	Brachydactyly	0011927	Short digit
6-9	Supernumerary digit　多指趾	0000562	Polydactyly	0010442	Polydactyly
6-10	Absent claw　爪欠損	0008494	Absence of all nails	0001817	Absent fingernail
6-11	Small claw　爪小型化	0012399	Short nails	0001804	Hypoplastic fingernail
7-1	Absent tail　無尾	0003456	Absent tail		
7-2	Bent tail　屈曲尾	0000585	Kinked tail		
7-3	Bifurcated tail　二又尾	0013175	Bifurcated tail		
7-4	Curled tail　巻いた尾	0003051	Curly tail		
7-5	Fleshy tab tail　尾付属物	0013177	Abnormal tail tip morphology		
7-6	Hooked tail　カギ状尾	0002111	Abnormal tail morphology		
7-7	Kiked tail　曲尾	0003051	Curly tail		
7-8	Misshapen tail　尾形態異常	0002111	Abnormal tail morphology		
7-9	Narrow tail　狭窄尾	0000589	Thin tail		
7-10	Short tail　短尾	0000592	Short tail		
7-11	Thread-like tail　索状尾	0002632	Vestigial tail		
8-1	Absent anus　肛門欠損	0003130	Anal atresia	0002023	Anal atresia
8-2	Small anus　肛門小型	0009052	Anal stenosis	0002025	Anal stenosis
8-3	Externalized heart　心臓逸所	0011660	Ectopia cordis	0001683	Ectopia cordis
8-4	Gastroschisis　腹壁裂	0000757	Herniated abdominal wall	0001543	Gastroschisis
8-6	Hypospadias　尿道下裂			0000047	Hypospadias
8-7	Holorachischisis　完全脊椎裂	0008784	Craniorachischisis		
8-8	Spina bifida　二分脊椎裂	0003054	Spina bifida	0002414	Spina bifida
8-9	Thoracogastroschisis　胸腹壁裂	0000757	Herniated abdominal wall	0100656	Thoracoabdominal wall defects
8-10	Small trunk　短躯	0001258	Decreased body length	0003521	Disproportionate short-trunk short stature
8-11	Omphalocele　臍帯ヘルニア	0003052	Omphalocele	0001539	Omphalocele
8-12	Umbilical hernia　臍ヘルニア	0010146	Umbilical hernia	0001537	Umbilical hernia

MP: Mouse phenotype
HP: Human phenotype
In some cases, MP and HP terms indicate a more general description for the Atlas term.

Photographs of Normal Fetuses in Rats, Rabbits and Mice
正常写真（ラット、ウサギ、マウス）

Rats

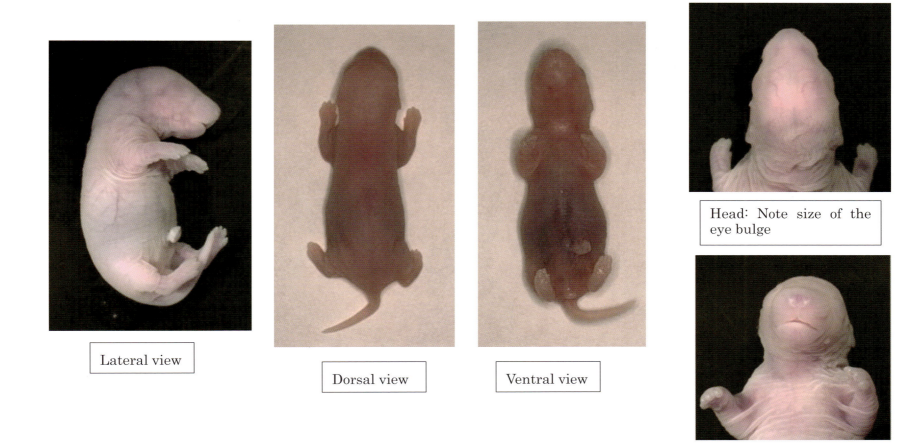

Lateral view

Dorsal view

Ventral view

Head: Note size of the eye bulge

Rats (continued)

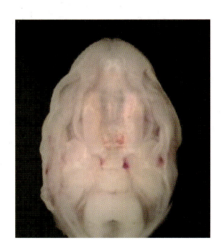

Palate

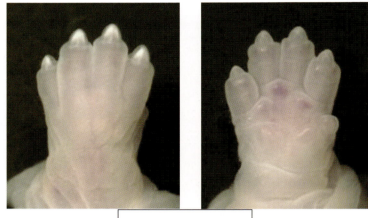

Digit (Fore-paw)

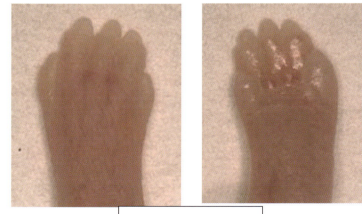

Digit (Hind-paw)

Rabbits (Kbl:NZW)

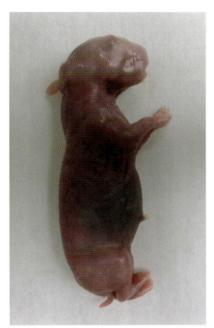
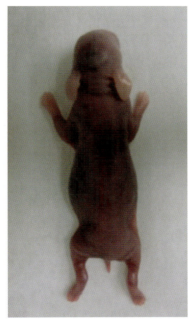
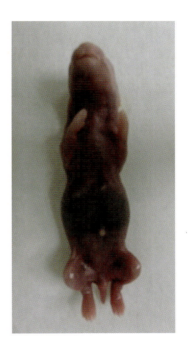
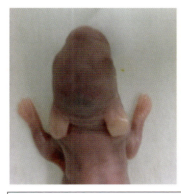
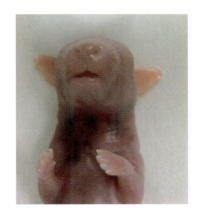

Lateral view

Dorsal view

Ventral view

Head: Note size of the eye bulge

Rabbits (continued)

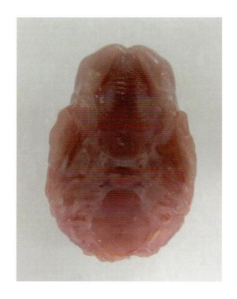

Palate

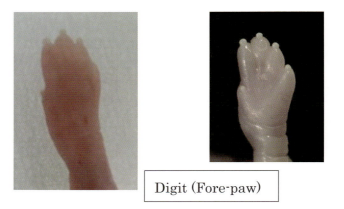

Digit (Fore-paw)

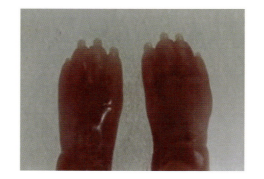

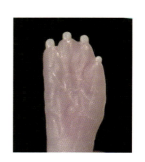

Digit (Hind-paw)

Mice (Crj:CD)

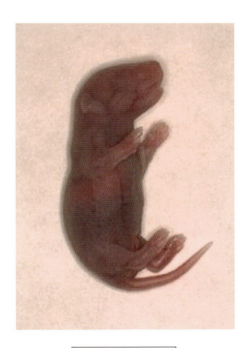

Lateral view

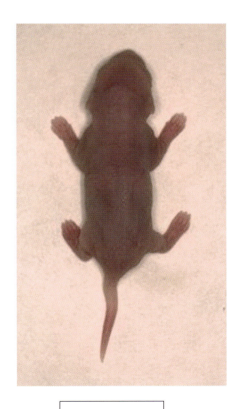

Dorsal view

Mice (continued)

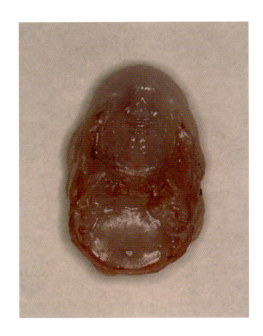

Palate

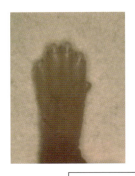 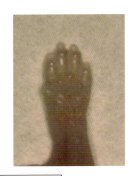

Digit (Fore-paw)

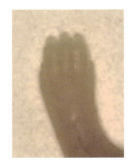 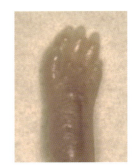

Digit (Hind-paw)

Photographs of External Anomalies

1. General

1-1 Generalized subcutaneous edema, Anasarca　全身性皮下浮腫　(Code No.: 10001, MP No.: 0011738, HP No.: 0012050)

Species	Rat
Memo	Generalized subcutaneous edema, Anasarca: An accumulation of interstitial fluid is observed in subcutaneous connective tissue. In the example shown, it is prominent between the lower jaw and forelimbs.
	全身性皮下浮腫、全身性浮腫：皮下結合組織における間質液の貯留により、全身に皮下浮腫がみられる。特に下顎と前肢の間が顕著。

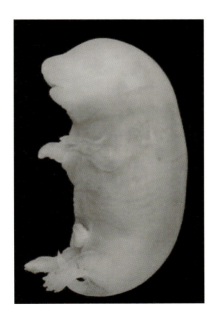
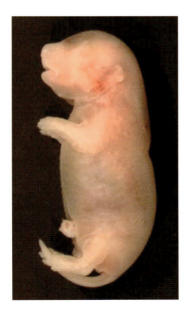
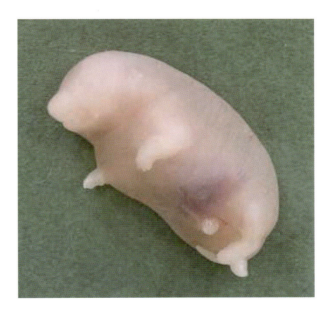

1-2　Conjoined twins　二重体（Code No.: 10002）

Conjoined twins, or omphalosite	Twins, originating from the same fertilized egg, with variable incomplete or complete separation into two during cleavage or early stages of embryogenesis: The completely separated fetuses are "Monozygotic twins" and the incompletely separated fetuses are "Conjoined twins". The conjoined twins are divided to two types; one is symmetrically joined and another is asymmetrically joined. The former is classified by the point at which their bodies are joined such as Craniopagus, Thoracopagus, Thoraco-omphalopagus, and Omphalopagus, etc. The latter is also called "Parasitic twins" or "Fetus in fetus" because they are joined asymmetrically. In the examples shown below, conjoined twin fetuses with duplicated limbs, tails, and external genitalia are observed.
二重体	1個の受精卵が卵割あるいは胚発生の早い時期に種々の程度で完全あるいは不完全に2つに分かれたものを言う。それぞれ個体として完全に分離しているものを**一卵性双生児**、2つの個体が連絡しているものを**結合体（二重体、Conjoined twins）**と言う。結合体は**対称性結合体（二重体）**と**非対称性結合体（二重体）**に分類される。**対称性二重体**は、それぞれの個体が均等に発生・発育したもので、結合面を軸として対称的に結合し、結合部位により、頭蓋結合体、頭胸結合体、胸腹結合体、殿結合体、二頭体など様々な結合体に分類される。**非対称性二重体**は2つの個体の発生・発育が異なるもので、良く発育した個体を自生体（Autosite）、発育の悪い個体を寄生体（Parasite）と言い、寄生的頭蓋結合体、寄生的胸結合体、仙骨部結合体など様々な結合体に分類される。また、完全に発達した児（自生体）内で不完全な胎児（寄生体）が発育しているもの（所謂、胎児内胎児、Fetus in fetus）まで様々な結合状態がある。四肢や尾・外部生殖器など一部の構造のみ重複している場合もある。

1-2 Continued

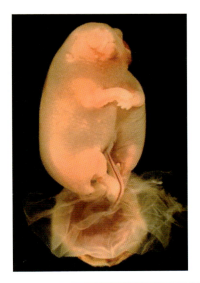
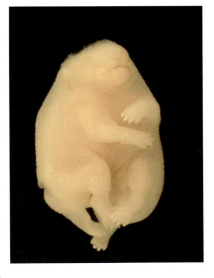

Species	Rat
Memo	Conjoined twins: Two fetuses fuse from head to abdomen.
	二重体：対称性結合体、頭部から胸腹部にかけ結合している。

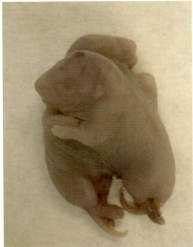

Species	Rat, Crl:CD(SD)
Memo	Conjoined twins: Two fetuses fuse at the thoracic and abdominal regions.
	二重体：対称性結合体、胸腹部で結合している。

1-2   Continued

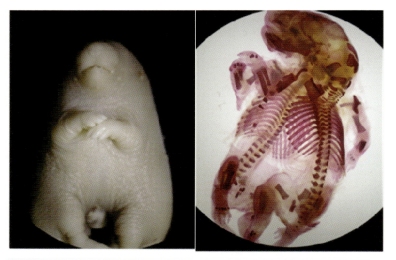

Species	Rat
Memo	Conjoined twins, Cranio-thoraco-omphalopagus: Photograph of the skeletal specimen from the twins (Double vertebral canal: Code No. New) is attached.
	二重体：頭部・胸部・腹部結合体、参考に本例の骨格写真（脊柱管二重、Code No. New) も添付する。

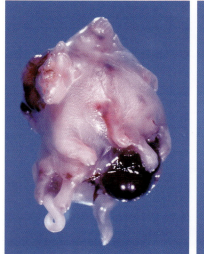
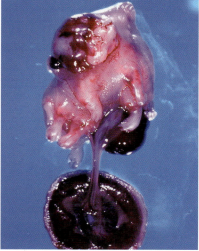

Species	Rat, Crl:CD(SD)
Memo	Conjoined twins (triplet): 3 sets of limbs are observed in the twins.
	三重体：四肢が３体分重複している

1-2 Continued

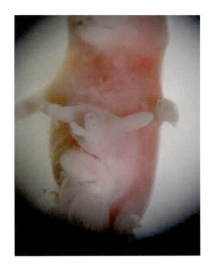

Species	Rat, SD (Dead fetus)
Memo	Conjoined twins: A parasite, that is mainly hind limbs, is observed in the abdomen. These fetuses are classified as "Fetus in fetus".
	二重体：非対称性結合体、腹部に後肢を主とする寄生体が認められる。胎児内胎児とも言われる。

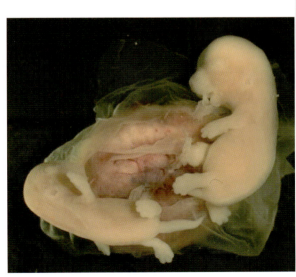 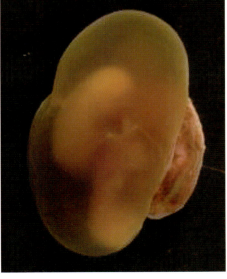

Species	Rat (Dead fetus)
Memo	Monozygotic twins: Two completely separated fetuses sharing one placenta.
	一卵性双生児：完全に分離した２匹の胎児が１つの胎盤を共有している。

1-2 Continued

The following specimens are considered to be possibly "Conjoined twins".

以下の標本も二重体（結合体）の一種と考える。

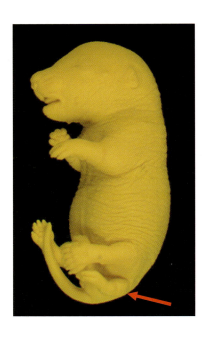

Species	Rat
Memo	Duplicated hind limb: Additional left limb is observed (arrow). The normal left limb has Polydactyly (10088).
	後肢重複：非対称性結合体の一種、左後肢が２本存在する。正常な後肢には多趾（10088）がみられる。

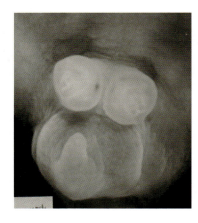

Species	Rat
Memo	Duplicated penis or Misshapen genital tubercle: This may be Conjoined twins with two genital tubercles.
	外生殖器形態異常（New）、重複外生殖器：対称性結合体の一種で、外生殖器が２個存在する。

1-2 Continued

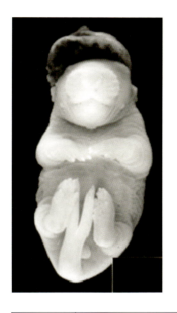 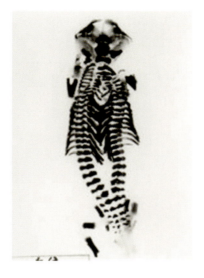

Species	Rat
Memo	Bifurcated tail (10097) with Exencephaly (10013): This may be conjoined twins. The photograph on the right shows, the skeletal specimen of this fetus, demonstrating Double vertebral canal (New).
	二又尾（10097）：対称性結合体の一種で、尾が中央付近から２本に分かれている。外脳（10013）を伴っている。右写真は本胎児の骨格標本であり、二重脊柱管（New）が確認できる。外表では観察できないが、全身的な二重体である。

Species	Rat
Memo	Bifurcated tail (10097): This may be conjoined twins with Exencephaly (10013). Although there is no skeletal specimen for this fetus, it may have Double vertebral canal (New) because of its wide body and V-typed line at the thoracic wall.
	二又尾（10097）、重複尾：対称性結合体の一種で、尾が２本存在する。外脳（10013）を伴っている。本胎児の骨格標本はないが、身体の太さおよび胸壁のV字型の影から、二重脊柱管（New）の可能性がある。

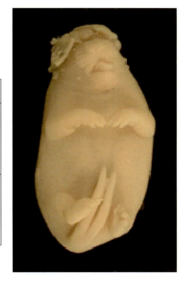

1-3 Subcutaneous hemorrhage 皮下出血 (Code No.: 10004, MP No.: 0011514, HP No.: 0001933)

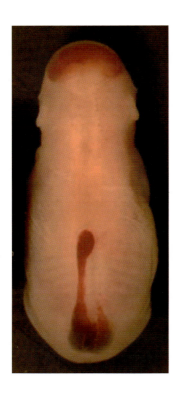

Species	Rat
Memo	Subcutaneous hemorrhage: Hemorrhage is observed at the head and back regions.
	皮下出血：頭部および背部に出血がみられる。

1-4　Absent skin　皮膚欠損　(Code No.: 10003, MP No.: 0003941, HP No.: 0001057)

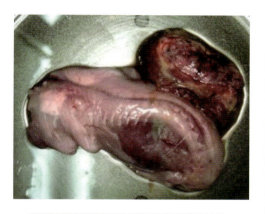

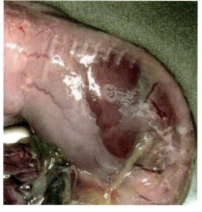

Species	Rabbit, NZW
Memo	Absent skin, Cutis aplasia: The skin of the whole body did not develop. Acephaly (10009) and Gastroschisis (10109) are also observed in this fetus. This fetus also has a finding similar to the "Amniotic band syndrome" described in human.
	皮膚欠損、皮膚無形成：全身の皮膚が形成されていない。無頭症（10009），腹壁裂（10109）を伴う。 ヒトでのamniotic band syndrome（羊膜索症候群）に類似している（羊膜や臍帯が付着している場合）。

1-5　Skin tag　皮膚付属物　(Code No.: New, MP No.: 0009931, HP No.: 0010609)

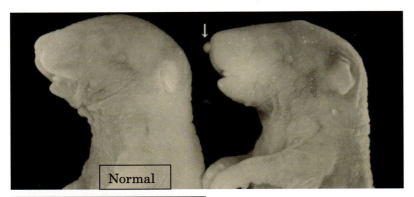

Species	Mouse
Memo	Skin tag around the nose : Small appendage of skin at the tip of the nose.
	皮膚付属物：鼻先端付近に小さな付属物。

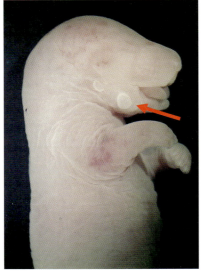

Species	Rat
Memo	Skin tag at the lower jaw : Small appendage of skin attached to the lower jaw.
	皮膚付属物：下顎に小さな付属物。

1-5 Continued

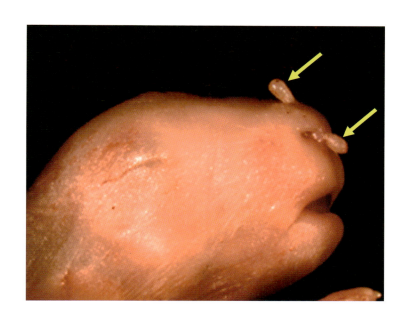

Species	Rabbit, Kbl:JW
Memo	Skin tag around the nose : Small appendages of skin around the nose.
	皮膚付属物：鼻先端付近に小さな付属物。

Photographs of External Anomalies

2. Head and Neck

2-1　Acephalostomia　無頭有口　(Code No.: 10008)

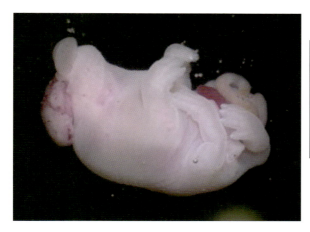

Species	Rat, Crl:CD(SD)
Memo	Acephalostomia: Absence of the head with a tongue-like structure. Exencephaly (10013), Gastroschisis (10109) and Short trunk (10117) are also observed.
	無頭有口：頭部の大部分が欠損しているが、舌が観察される。 外脳（10013）、腹壁裂（10109）、短躯（10117）を伴っている。

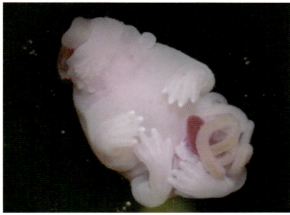

2-1 Continued

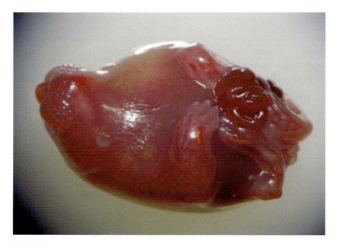

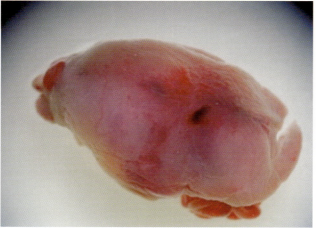

Species	Rat, Crl:CD(SD)
Memo	Acephalostomia: Absence of the head with a mouth-like orifice. Anencephaly (10010), Gastroschisis (10109) and Short trunk (10117) are also observed.
	無頭有口：頭部の大部分が欠損しているが、舌（口の様な孔）が観察される。無脳（10010）、腹壁裂（10109）、短躯（10117）を伴っている。

2-2 Cranioschisis 頭蓋裂 (Code No.: 10011, MP No.: 0000919)

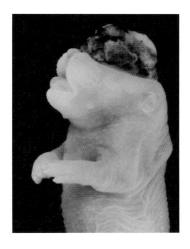

Species	Rat
Memo	Cranioschisis: The brain is exposed by fissure of the cranial region of the head.
	頭蓋裂：頭蓋部位の裂により脳が露出している。

2-3　Exencephaly　外脳　(Code No.: 10013, MP No.: 0000914)

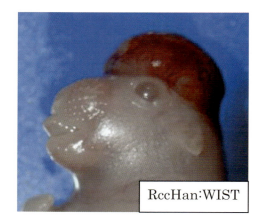
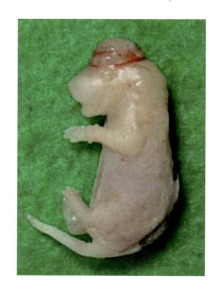

Species	Rat
Memo	Exencephaly with Open eye (10033)
	外脳：眼開存（Open eye、10033）を伴うことが多い。

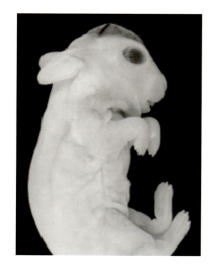

Species	Rabbit
Memo	Exencephaly with Open eye (10033) and Hyperflexion of forepaws (10087).
	外脳：眼開存（10033）及び過屈曲手（10087）も伴う。

2-3 Continued

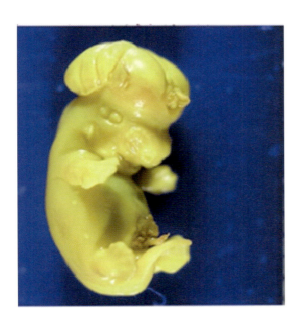

Species	Mouse, ICR
Memo	Exencephaly: Fetus on day 15 of gestation
	外脳：妊娠15日の胎児。

2-4　Absent head　頭部欠損　(Code No.: 10009, MP No.: 0009579)

Species	Rabbit
Memo	Absent head, Acephaly: Absence of the head
	頭部欠損、無頭（症）：頭部が欠損している。左の胎児では、舌など一部の頭部・顔面組織がみられるが、頭部の大部分が欠損しており、頭部欠損（無頭）の範疇とする。

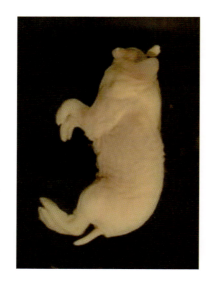
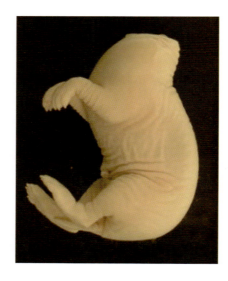

2-5 Domed head　ドーム状頭部　(Code No.: 10012, MP No.: 0000440)

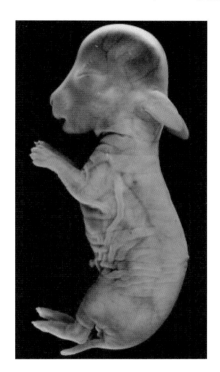

Species	Rabbit
Memo	Domed head: Cranial region of head appears more elevated and rounded than normal. Pay attention when performing visceral examination because this may be associated with "Hydrocephaly".
	ドーム状頭部：頭蓋が異常に高い。水頭を伴う場合があり、内臓検査時には注意する。

2-6 Cranial meningocele 頭蓋髄膜瘤 (Code No.: 10016, MP No.: 0012259, HP No.: 0002435)

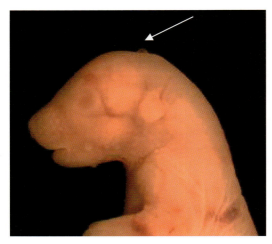

Species	Rat
Memo	Cranial meningocele: Herniation of meninges through a defect in skull. This is different from Meningoencephalocele (10017) which has herniation of brain and meninges.
	頭蓋髄膜瘤：頭蓋骨欠損により髄膜のみ突出している。髄膜脳瘤（10017）は脳及び髄膜の突出であり、区分する。

2-7 Meningo-encephalocele 髄膜脳瘤 (Code No.: 10017, MP No.: 0012260, HP No.: 0002084)

Species	Mouse and Rat
Memo	Herniation of **brain** and **meninges** through a cranial opening. This finding is different from "Cranial meningocele" which only shows herniation of **meninges**.
	頭蓋の開口により、**脳**及び**髄膜**が突出している。皮膚に被われている場合もあり、頭部の局所的な隆起などに注意する。その際、頭部割面の観察で確認する。**髄膜**のみのヘルニアは「頭蓋髄膜瘤（10016）」であり、本所見とは区分する。

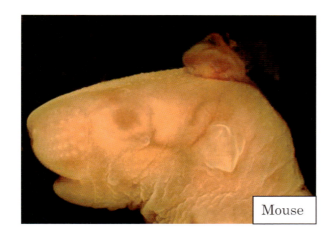

Mouse

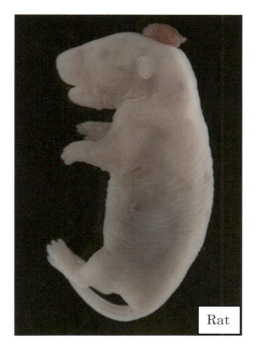

Rat

2-8 Meningohydro-encephalocele 髄膜水脳瘤 (Code No.: New)

Species	Rat, Wistar/SD
Memo	Meningohydro-encephalocele: Herniation of brain, cerebral ventricle, and meninges through a defect in skull. This is different from "Meningo-encephalocele" which is herniation of brain and meninges.
	髄膜水脳瘤：頭蓋欠損による脳、脳室及び髄膜のヘルニア。頭部割面の観察で確認する必要がある。「髄膜脳瘤（10017）」は脳と髄膜のヘルニアであり、区分する。

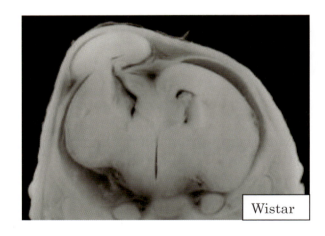
Wistar

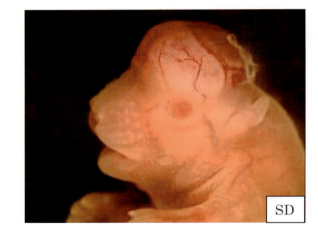
SD

Photographs of External Anomalies

3. Ear and Eye

3-1 Malpositioned pinna　耳介位置異常　(Code No.: 10021, MP No.: 0000023, HP No.: 0000357)

Species	Rat, Wistar
Memo	Malpositioned pinna, Low set pinna (arrows); This is "Otocephaly" caracterized by absence or severe hypoplasia of lower jaws and low-set pinna.
	耳介位置異常、耳介低位：本例は下顎の欠損あるいは著しい形成不全と耳介低位を特徴とする典型的な耳頭症と考えられる。

Right photograph: Skeletal specimen
Skeletal specimen of a fetus with low-set pinna: Malpositioned tympanic annulus (arrow) with Small (10470) and Fused (10467) mandible; Tympanic annulus is located near the center of the skull. This anomaly is usually observed in a fetus with malpositioned auricle or pinna (Otocephaly).
耳介位置異常の骨格標本：耳介の低位に伴い、鼓室輪が中央に寄っている。下顎骨の小型（10470）及び癒合（10467）も伴う典型的な「耳頭症」の例。

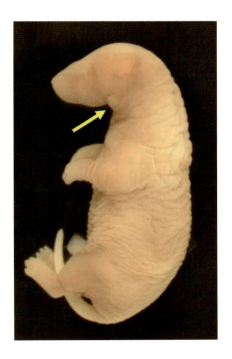
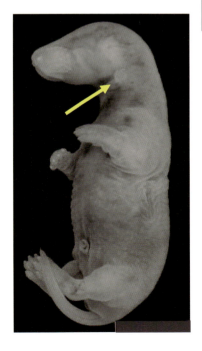
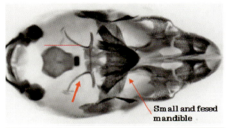
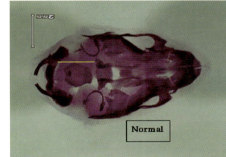

3-2 Small pinna, Microtia 耳介小型（化）(Code No.: 10022, MP No.: 0000018, HP No.: 0008551)

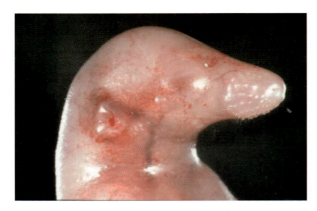

Species	Rat
Memo	Microtia, small external ear with Agnathia (absent lower jaw, 10047)
	小耳、小耳介：耳介が小さい。無顎（10047）を伴う。

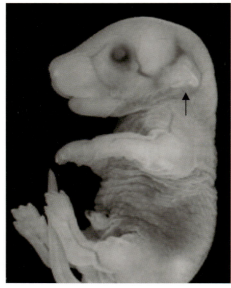

Species	Mouse, yellow KK
Memo	Microtia (arrow)
	小耳、小耳介

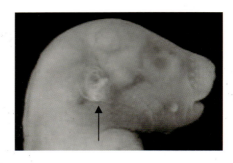

Species	Rat
Memo	Microtia (arrow)
	小耳、小耳介

3-3 Cyclopia 単眼 (Code No.: 10027, MP No.: 0005163, HP No.: 0009914)

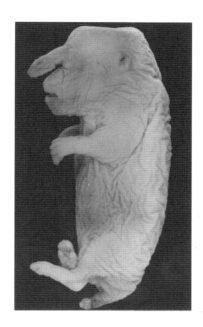

Species	Rat
Memo	Cyclopia: Single median orbit, eyeballs are completely fused, and snout appears as a frontonasal appendage (Proboscis, 10043) above the orbit.
	単眼：単一の眼窩（眼球）が完全に癒合している。眼窩の上に象鼻（10043）が確認される。象鼻を伴う場合は「長鼻単眼症」とも言われる。

Species	Rabbit
Memo	Cyclopia: Single median orbit, eyeballs are completely fused, and snout appears as a frontonasal appendage (Proboscis, 10043) above the orbit. Maxilla (upper jaw) is small (10060).
	単眼：単一の眼窩（眼球）が完全に癒合している。眼窩の上に象鼻（10043）が確認される。上顎小型（10060）も伴う。「長鼻単眼症」とも言われる。

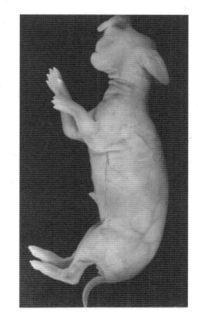

3-3 Continued

Species	Rat
Memo	Cyclopia: Single median orbit, eyeballs are completely fused, and snout appears as a frontonasal appendage (Proboscis, 10043) above the orbit. Maxilla (upper jaw) is small (10060).
	単眼：単一の眼窩（眼球）が完全に癒合している。眼窩の上に象鼻（10043）が確認される。上顎小型（10060）も伴う。

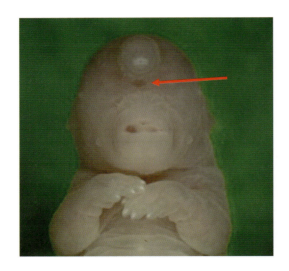
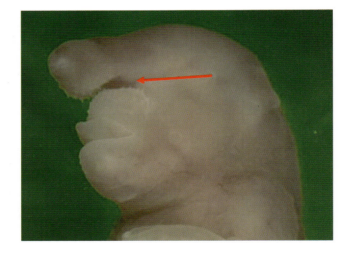

3-3 Continued

Species	Rat
Memo	Cyclopia: Eyeballs are completely fused, and Proboscis (10043) and Astomia (absent mouth, 10050) are observed. Hypogenesis of the head and face is also observed. The skeletal specimen of this fetus is also shown.
	単眼：単一の眼が確認できる。象鼻（10043）、無口（10050）も確認できる。「長鼻単眼症」とも言われる。全般的な頭部の形成不全を伴う。参考に本胎児の骨格写真も添付する。

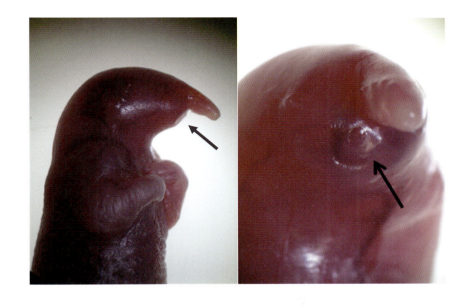

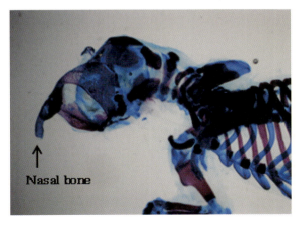

3-4　Open eye　眼開存　(Code No.: 10033, MP No.: 0001302)

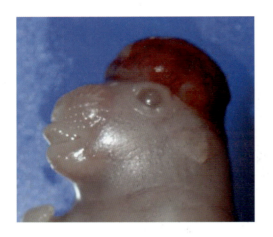

Species	Rat, RccHan:WIST
Memo	Open eye with Exencephaly (10013), Short lower jaw (10058), and Short upper jaw (10060): Open eye often occurs in a fetus with Exencephaly.
	眼開存：本所見は外脳（10013）を持つ胎児に良く発現する。上下顎の小型化（10058 および 10060）も伴う。

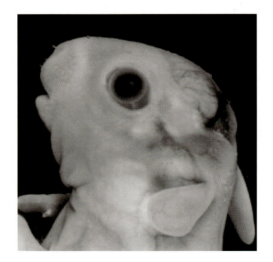

Species	Rabbit
Memo	Open eye with Cranioschisis (10011)
	眼開存：頭蓋裂（10011）を伴う。

3-5   Protruding eye, Exophthalmia   眼突出   (Code No.: 10029, MP No.: 0002750, HP No.: 0000520)

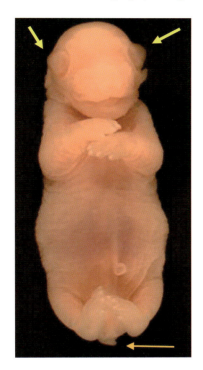

Species	Rat
Memo	Protruding eye, Exophthalmia with Short tail (10103): Excessive protrusion of the eye ball. Open eye (10033) also appears bilaterally.
	眼突出：眼球が過度に突出している。短尾（10103）および眼開存（10033）を伴う。骨格観察の場合、眼窩周囲の骨格形態に注意する。

3-6　Small eye bulge　眼部隆起扁平　(Code No.: 10035)

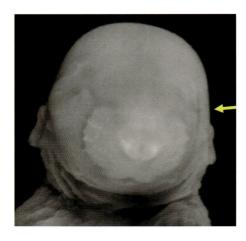

Species	Rat
Memo	Small eye bulge: This can be detected easily by looking down directly from above the head. Absent eye (10137) or Small eye (10143) should be confirmed in visceral examination when the specimen is a mouse or rat fetuse.
	眼部隆起扁平（化）：左眼の隆起がほとんどない。頭頂部から観察すると判断し易い。無眼球（内臓異常、10137）あるいは小眼球（内臓異常、10143）の場合があり、マウス、ラットの場合、内臓観察時に確認する。

3-7 Eyelid fissure, Open eyelid　眼瞼裂　(Code No.: 10034)

Species	Mouse, Rat, Rabbit
Memo	Eyelid fissure, Palpebral coloboma, (Open eyelid): A part of the eyelid is not fused. Note: This is different from "Open eye (10033)".
	眼瞼裂、眼瞼コロボーマ、(眼瞼開裂)、(眼瞼開存)：胎児期に癒合すべき眼瞼の一部が癒合していない。眼開存（10033）と区分する。

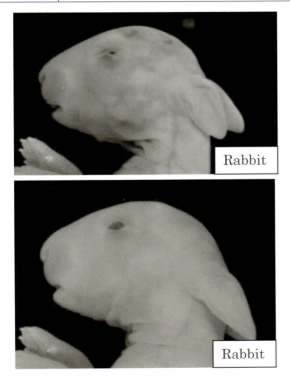

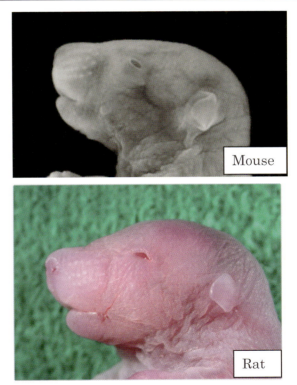

Photographs of External Anomalies

4. Face

4-1 Cleft face 顔面裂 (Code No.: 10036, MP No.: 0008797, HP No.: 0002006)

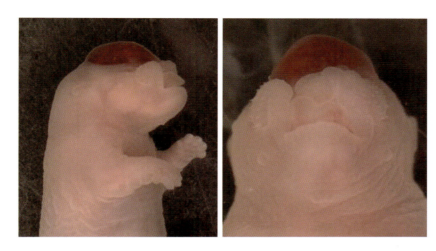

Species	Rat
Memo	Cleft face with Cranioschisis (10011). Fissure of face. This Cleft face also includes Cleft lip (10051)
	顔面裂：頭蓋裂（10011）を伴い、唇裂（10051）を含む顔面裂。顔面裂は、顔面及び顎の癒合の異常によって顔面に裂が生じた状態であり、重度の場合、頭部の形態異常も併発する。

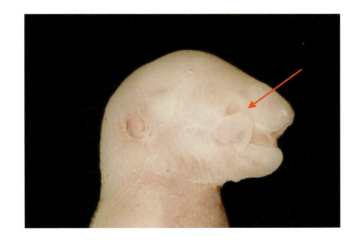

Species	Rat
Memo	Cleft face: Fissure is observed at the right upper jaw. It is also considered to be "Cleft upper jaw (New)".
	顔面裂。右上顎に裂がみられる。上顎裂（New）でも良い。

4-2 Absent lower jaw, Agnathia 無顎 (Code No.: 10047, MP No.: 0000087, HP No.: 0009939)

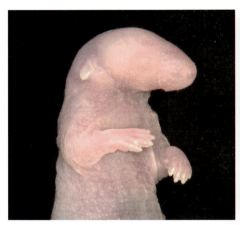
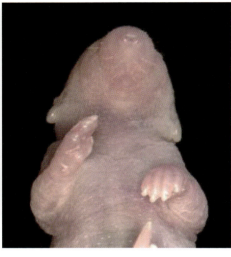

Species	Mouse, Crlj: CD1 (ICR)
Memo	Agnathia with Astomia (Absent mouth, 10050)
	無顎：無口（10050）を伴う。

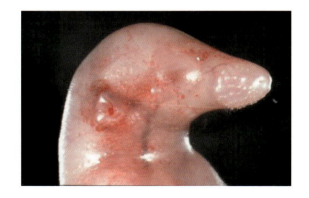

Species	Rat
Memo	Agnathia, absence of mandible (lower jaw) with Microtia (Small pinna, 10022)
	無顎、無下顎：下顎がほぼ欠損している。耳介の小型化（小耳介、小耳、10022）を伴っている。

4-2 Continued

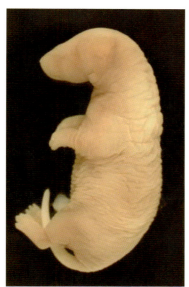

Species	Rat, Wistar
Memo	Agnathia, Absent lower jaw: This is "Otocephaly" caracterized by absence or severe hypoplasia of lower jaws and low-set pinna located at or near the midline.
	下顎欠損：本例は下顎の欠損あるいは著しい形成不全と耳介低位を特徴とする典型的な耳頭症と考えられる。

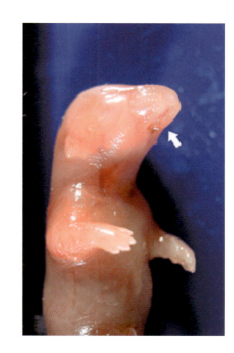

Species	Rat, Wistar Hannover
Memo	Agnathia, Absence of mandible (lower jaw): Almost all lower jaw is absent, and lip at the lower jaw is not observed.
	無顎：下顎がほぼ欠損し、口唇（下顎）もみられない。

4-3 Split/cleft mandible, Gnathoschisis　下顎裂　(Code No.: 10056, MP No.: 0000114, HP No.: 0010752)

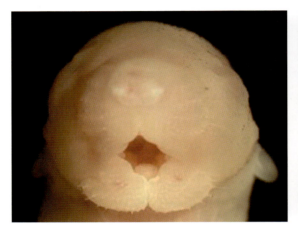
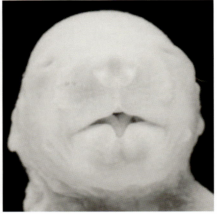

Species	Rat
Memo	Gnathoschisis or Split/cleft mandible
	下顎裂：下顎が正中で癒合していない。

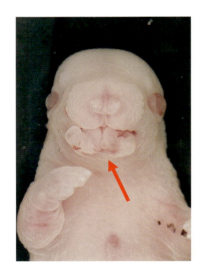

Species	Rat
Memo	Gnathoschisis or Split/cleft mandible with Open eye (10033)
	下顎裂：下顎が正中で癒合せず、開放性の裂（形態異常）がみられ、顔面裂（10036）の一種とも判断できる。眼開存（10033）もみられる。

4-3 Continued

Species	Rat, Wistar Hannover
Memo	Gnathoschisis or Split/cleft mandible: The right and left sides of the mandible did not fuse, and opened mandible was observed.
	下顎裂：下顎が正中で癒合せず、開放性の裂がみられる。

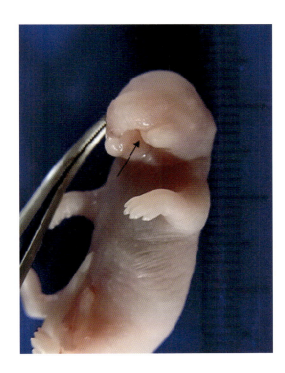

4-4 Small mandible, Micromandible, Brachygnathia 下顎小型（化）

(Code No.: 10058, MP No.: 0002639 or 0004592, HP No.: 0000347)

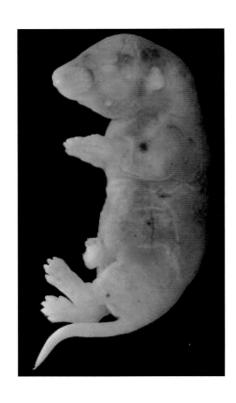

Species	Rat
Memo	Brachygnathia, Micromandible, Short lower jaw with Small head/Microcephaly (10018) at the occipital region of the head.
	小顎、小下顎、下顎短小：小頭（後頭部分、10018）もみられる。

4-4 Continued

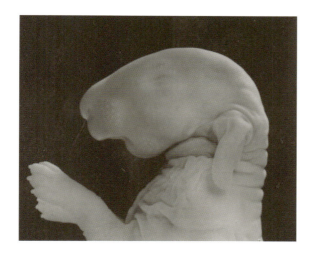

Species	Rabbit
Memo	Brachygnathia, Micromandible, or Short lower jaw
	小顎、小下顎、下顎短小

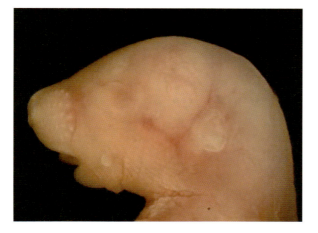

Species	Rat
Memo	Brachygnathia, Micromandible, or Short lower jaw
	小顎、小下顎、下顎短小

4-5　Cleft maxilla　上顎裂　(Code No.: New, MP No.: 0000455, HP No.: 0000326)

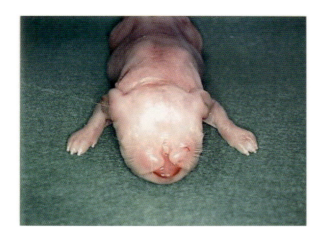

Species	Rabbit
Memo	Split maxilla, Gnathoschisis or Cleft maxilla: This is also "Cleft face (10036)" because fissure occurs at the center of the upper jaw and the shape of the nose is unclear.
	上顎裂：上顎の正中に裂が生じ、鼻の形態が確認し難いので、顔面裂（10036）でも良い。

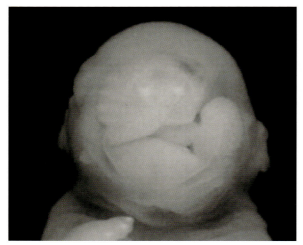

Species	Rat
Memo	Gnathoschisis or Split maxilla: Split at the upper jaw. This finding is more adverse than a Cleft lip (10051).
	上顎裂、顎裂：左上顎に裂がみられる。唇裂（10051）に比べ重度である。

4-6 Small upper jaw (maxilla), Maxillary micrognathia, Micromaxilla　上顎小型

(Code No.: 10060, MP No.: 0004540, HP No.: 0000327)

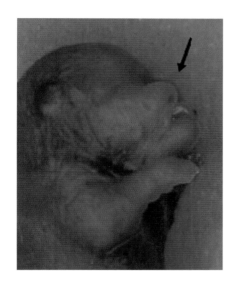

Species	Rat
Memo	Maxillary micrognathia with Misshapen snout (10041)
	小上顎：鼻形態異常（10041）を伴う。本例では上顎から前頭部にかけ、著しい形成不全が認められる。骨格あるいは脳の観察には注意を要する。

4-7 Cleft lip 唇裂 (Code No.: 10051, MP No.: 0005170, HP No.: 0000204)

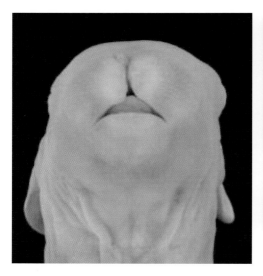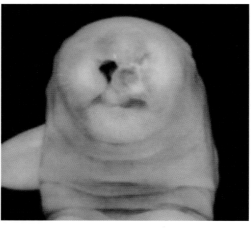

Species	Rabbit
Memo	Cleft lip: Fissure of the upper lip at the center or at a lateral location.
	唇裂：上唇の中央あるいは左右に裂がみられる。口蓋裂（10052）を伴うこともある。

4-8 Absent mouth, Astomia 無口 (Code No.: 10050, MP No.: 0000453, HP No.: 0000153)

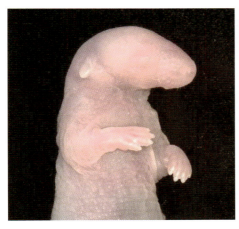 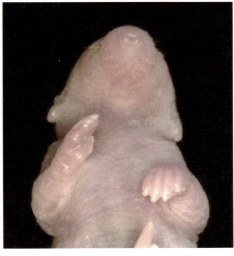

Species	Mouse, Crlj: CD1 (ICR)
Memo	Astomia with Agnathia (Absent lower jaw, 10047)
	無口：無顎（10047）を伴う。

4-9　Large mouth, Macrostomia　巨口　(Code No.: 10055, MP No.: 0009881, HP No.: 0000154)

Species	Rat
Memo	Macrostomia or Wide mouth with Large tongue (10054) or Protruding tongue (10065)
	巨口：正常例に比べ、口裂がより深く切れ込んでいる。舌先端と上下顎先端の位置関係から、舌の大型化（巨舌、10054）あるいは舌突出（10065）も伴うと思われる。

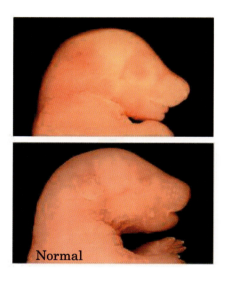
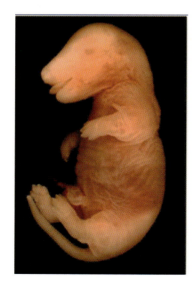

4-10 Cleft palate 口蓋裂 (Code No.: 10052, MP No.: 0000111, HP No.: 0000175)

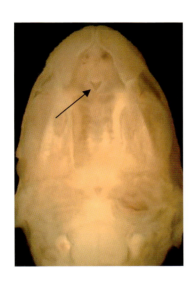

Species	Rat
Memo	Cleft palate, Partial cleft palate or Open incisive foramen (arrow): This anomaly can be detected/confirmed by using stereo-microscope or reexamination in the visceral examination.
	口蓋裂、**先端口蓋裂**、切歯孔開存とも言う。一次口蓋の発生異常あるいは一次口蓋と二次口蓋の接する部分の癒合不全により孔が残る。非常に観察し難い所見であり、実体顕微鏡による観察、あるいは、内臓観察時の再確認が望まれる。

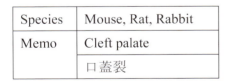

Species	Mouse, Rat, Rabbit
Memo	Cleft palate
	口蓋裂

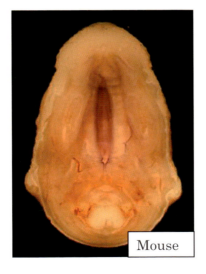
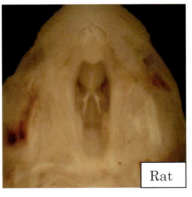
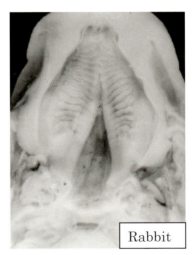

4-11　Misaligned palatal rugae　口蓋ヒダ不整列　(Code No.: 10063, MP No.: 0009652, HP No.: 0000174)

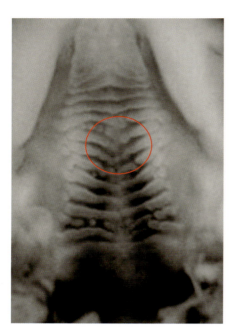

Species	Rabbit
Memo	Misaligned palatal rugae: Asymmetrically aligned and irregular palatal rugae. This may also be "Misshapen palatal rugae (10064)". In the examination for mouse or rat fetuses, this anomaly can be detected by using stereo-microscope or reexamination in the visceral examination.
	口蓋ヒダ不整列：左右の口蓋ヒダがずれている。全体としては、不連続もみられ、「口蓋ヒダ形態異常（10064）」でも良い。マウスやラットの場合、口蓋は観察し難い部位であるため、実体顕微鏡による観察、あるいは、内臓観察時の再確認が望まれる。

4-12 Misshapen palatal rugae　口蓋ヒダ形態異常　(Code No.: 10064, MP No.: 0009652, HP No.: 0000174)

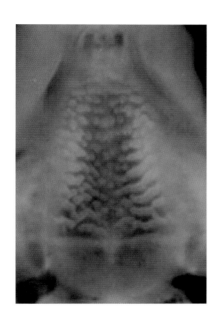

Species	Rabbit
Memo	Misshapen palatal rugae: Many rugae are not uniform and short. In the examination of mouse or rat fetuses, this anomaly can be detected by using stereo-microscope or reexamination in the visceral examination.
	口蓋ヒダ形態異常：口蓋ヒダが切断し、小さくなっている。マウスやラットの場合、口蓋は観察し難い部位であるため、実体顕微鏡による観察、あるいは、内臓観察時の再確認が望まれる。

4-13 Proboscis 象鼻 (Code No.: 10043, MP No.: 0006290, HP No.: 0012806)

Species	Rat
Memo	Proboscis: Tubular projection replaces the snout.
	象鼻：筒状の突起物がある。単眼（10027）の場合にもよくみられる。

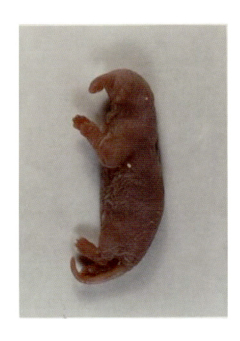
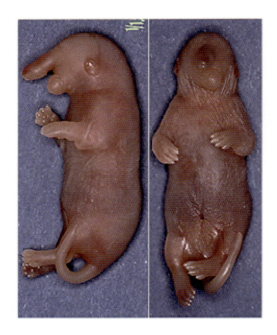

4-14 Misshapen snout 鼻形態異常 (Code No.: 10041, MP No.: 0002233, HP No.: 0005105)

Species	Rat
Memo	Misshapen snout (arrow) with short upper and lower jaw (10058, 10060)
	鼻形態異常：小上下顎 (10058, 10060)を伴う。

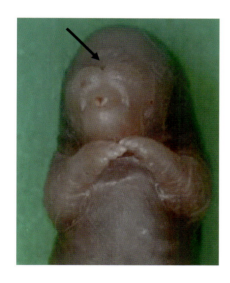
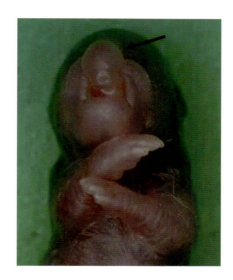

4-15 Protruding tongue 舌突出 (Code No.: 10065, MP No.: 0009908, HP No.: 0010808)

Species	Rat
Memo	Protruding tongue with Large tongue (Macroglossia, 10054) and Large mouth (Macrostomia, 10055), and with Kinked tail (10100) in the left fetus
	舌突出：舌先端と上下顎先端の位置関係から、舌が突出していると判断される。舌の大型化（巨舌、10054）も伴うと思われる。また、両写真の所見例共に口裂が正常例に比べより深く切れ込んでおり、口の大型化（巨口、10055）もみられる。左写真の胎児では曲尾（10100）もみられる。

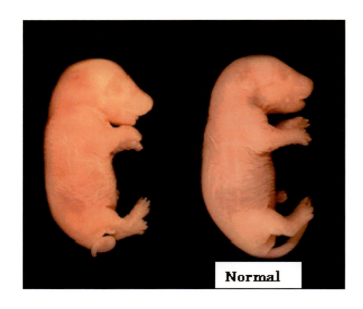

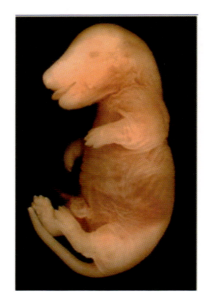

4-16　**Ankyloglossia**　舌癒合　(Code No.: 10048, MP No.: 0013264, HP No.: 0010296)

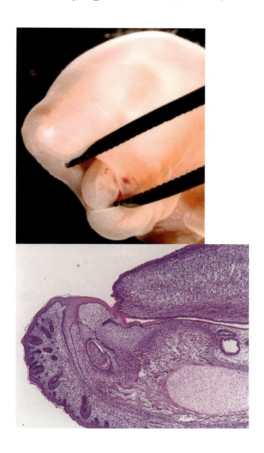

Species	Rat
Memo	Ankyloglossia: Tongue fused to floor of the mouth by hyper-growth of the tongue epithelium. Lower figure: histology of the specimen above.
	舌癒合：舌が口腔底部と癒合している。下図は上記写真の病理像（舌上皮の過形成による舌と口腔底部の癒合が確認できる）。

Photographs of External Anomalies

5. Limb

5-1   Absent limb, Amelia   無肢   (Code No.: 10066, MP No.: 0000549, HP No.: 0009827)

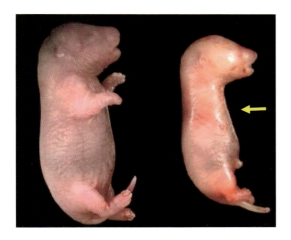
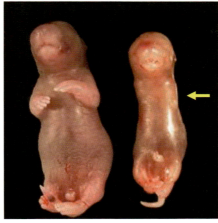

Species	Rat
Memo	Amelia (arrow): Complete absence of both forelimbs. Fetus at the left of each photograph is normal.
	無肢、欠肢：左右の前肢がほぼ欠損している。各左胎児は正常。

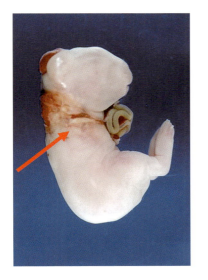

Species	Rabbit
Memo	Amelia with Exencephaly (10013), Short trunk (10117), Omphalocele (10115), and Anury (Absent tail, 10093): Complete absence of both forelimbs
	無肢、欠肢：左右の前肢がほぼ欠損している。外脳（10013）、短躯（10117）、臍帯ヘルニア（10115）、無尾（10093）を伴う。

5-2　Hyperextension of limb　過伸展肢　(Code No.: 10069, MP No.: 0002109, HP No.: 0005750)

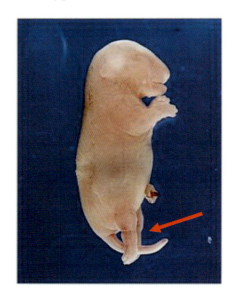

Species	Rat
Memo	Hyperextension of hindlimb: Both hindlimbs are over-extended (arrow).
	過伸展肢：両側の後肢が著しく伸びている。

Species	Cynomolgus monkey
Memo	Hyperextension of hindlimb: Right hindlimb ia over-extended (arrow).
	過伸展肢：右側の後肢が著しく伸びている。

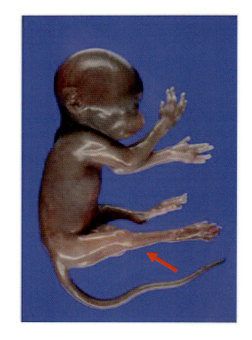

5-3　Malrotated limb　異常回転肢　(Code No.: 10072, MP No.: 0002109)

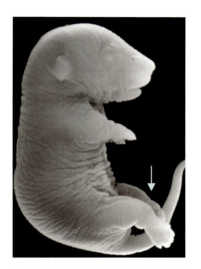

Species	Rat
Memo	Malrotated limb of the hindlimb: Hindlimb turned toward the midline (inward rotation). Forelimb is Micromelia (Brachymelia or Short limb, 10073).
	異常回転肢：後肢全体が中心（内側）に回転している。外側の場合もある。前肢は小肢（10073）骨格異常を伴うこともあり、骨格観察時には留意する。

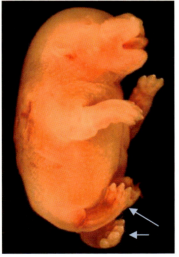

Species	Rat
Memo	Malrotated hindlimb: With Short trunk (10117), Misshapen head (New) and Anury (Absent tail, 10093)
	異常回転肢（後肢）：短躯（10117）、頭部形態異常（New）、無尾（10093）を伴う。骨格異常を伴うこともあり、骨格観察時には留意する。

5-3 Continued

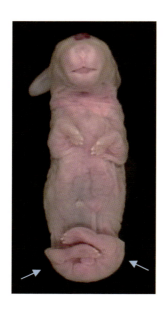

Species	Rabbit
Memo	Malrotated hindlimb with Hyperflecxion of the forelimb (Flexed forelimb, 10070)
	異常回転肢（後肢）：過屈曲手（前肢、10087）を伴う。骨格異常を伴うこともあり、骨格観察時には留意する。

5-4　Micromelia　小肢　(Code No.: 10073, MP No.: 0008736, HP No.: 0002983)

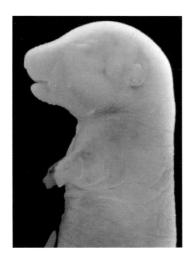

Species	Rat
Memo	Micromelia, Brachymelia, or Short forelimb: Note to compare with Hemimelia (10068, absence or shortening of the distal two segments of the limb.
	小肢、短肢：前肢全体が短い。半肢（10068、前腕と下腿あるいは手と足部分の欠損あるいは短小）と区分する。骨格異常を伴うので、骨格観察時には留意する。

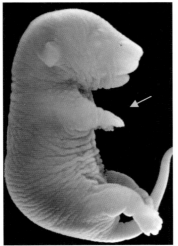

Species	Rat
Memo	Micromelia, Brachymelia, or Short forelimb: Note to compare with Hemimelia (10068, absence or shortening of the distal two segments of the limb). Hindlimb is Malrotated limb (10072)
	小肢、短肢：前肢全体が短い。半肢（10068、前腕と下腿あるいは手と足部分の欠損あるいは短小）と区分する。骨格異常を伴うので、骨格観察時には留意する。後肢は異常回転肢（10072）。

5-5　Phocomelia　フォコメリア　(Code No.: 10074, MP No.: 0002109, HP No.: 0009829)

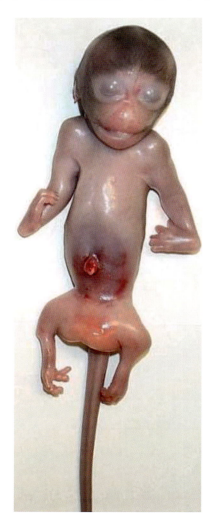

Species	Cynomolgus monkey
Memo	Phocomelia: Fetus treated with thalidomide 　Severe reduction of hindlimb and slight reduction of forelimb with Malrotated paw (Talipes, 10084) of forelimb.
	フォコメリア（サリドマイド投与） 下肢の減形成（小型化、短縮）、上肢上腕部の軽度短縮、異常回転手（内反手、10084）を合併。

5-5 Continued

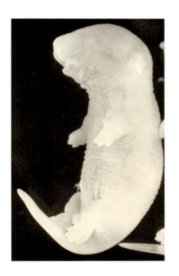

Species	Mouse
Memo	Ectromelia (absence or shortening of distal segment of limb) with Ectrodactyly (Oligodactyly) of fore- and hindlimbs : Reduction of proximal portion of fore- and hindlimbs
	フォコメリア：前肢、後肢とも短縮・小型化（減形成）：欠指、欠趾も伴っている。

Species	Rat
Memo	Phocomelia: Phocomelia in the forelimb and Micromelia (10073) and Polydactyly (10088) in the hindlimb
	フォコメリア：前肢はフォコメリア、後肢は小肢（10073）及び多趾（10088）。

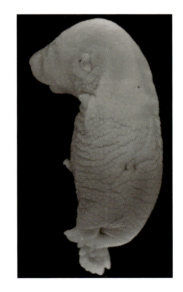

Photographs of External Anomalies

6. Paw and Digit

6-1   Absent digit, Adactyly   無指趾   (Code No.: 10077, MP No.: 0000561, HP No.: 0009776)

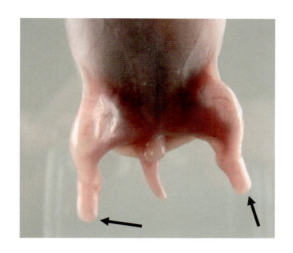

Species	Rabbit
Memo	Adactyly with Short tail (10103): Absence of all digits of both hind-paws
	無趾：両側の全趾が欠損している。短尾（10103）を伴う。

6-2 Few digit, Ectrodactyly, Oligodactyly 欠指趾 (Code No.: 10080, MP No.: 0005230, HP No.: 0100257)

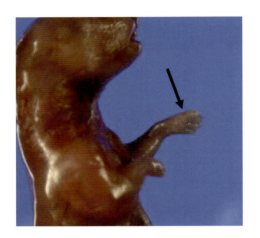

Species	Rabbit
Memo	Preaxial Ectrodactyly of fore-paw: Absence of the first digit
	前肢の軸前性欠指：第一指の欠損

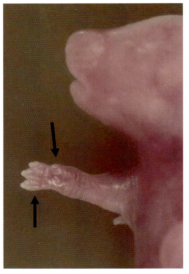

Species	Rat
Memo	Ectrodactyly (Oligodactyly) of fore-paw：Absent of the first digit and 1 other (possibly post-axial) digit; A careful skeletal examination of the specimens should be performed because it may be difficult to distinguish between Ectrodactyly and Syndactyly (10091) in external examination.
	欠指：第一指ともう１指（軸後性かも）。なお、合指（10091）との判別が難しい場合もあり、骨格観察時に留意する。

6-2 Continued

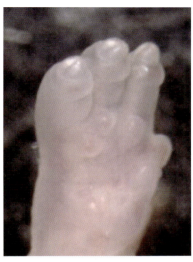

Species	Rat
Memo	Oligodactyly or Ectrodactyly of the fore-paw: Post-axial
	欠指、乏指：軸後性

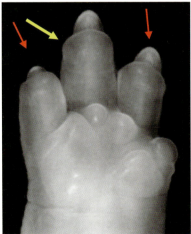

Species	Rat
Memo	Oligodactyly or Ectrodactyly: Axial Oligodactyly with Brachydactyly (10079, red arrow). A careful skeletal examination of the specimens should be performed because the 3rd digit (yellow arrow) is slightly enlarged and it may be difficult to distinguish between Ectrodactyly and Syndactyly (10091) in external examination.
	欠指、乏指：中軸性、短指（10079、赤矢印）も伴う。なお、第3指（黄色矢印）がやや太く、合指（10091）との判別が難しい場合もあり、骨格観察時に留意する。

6-3 Fused digit, Syndactyly 合指趾 (Code No.: 10091, MP No.: 0000564, HP No.: 0001159)

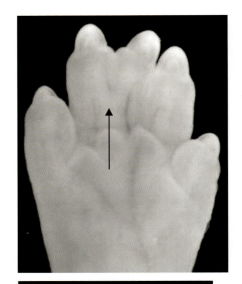
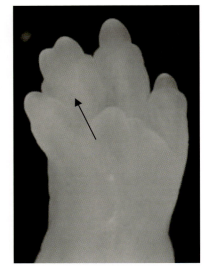

Species	Rat
Memo	Syndactyly of the hind-paw
	合趾

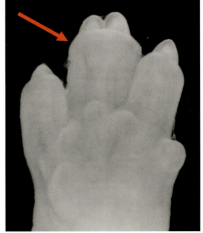
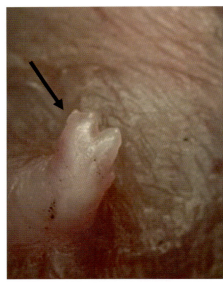

Species	Rat
Memo	Syndactyly of the fore-paw: The 3rd and 4th digits of fore-paw are fused.
	合指：第3及び4指の合指

Species	Rat
Memo	Syndactyly of the fore-paw
	合指

6-4 Large digit, Macrodactyly, Dactylomegaly　巨大指趾　(Code No.: 10081, MP No.: 0013149, HP No.: 0004099)

Species	Rat
Memo	Dactylomegaly, Macrodactyly or Megalodactyly of the hind-paw (arrow): Pre-axial Dactylomegaly with Polydactyly (10088) of the hind-paw (arrow).
	巨大趾：軸前性、軸前性多趾（10088）を伴う。

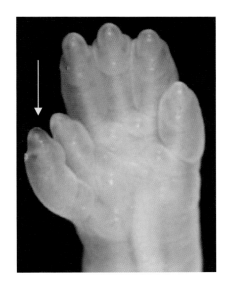
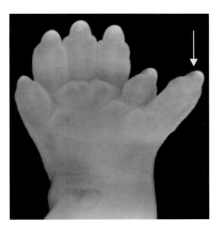

6-5 Malpositioned digit, Clinodactyly　指趾位置異常

(Code No.: 10083, MP No.: 0006253 or 0003807, HP No.: 0030084 or 0012385)

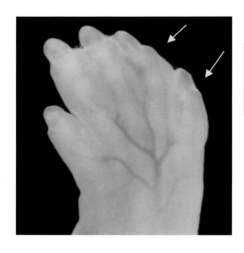

Species	Rat
Memo	Clinodactyly: Deflection of digits from the central axis
	斜趾：中心軸から趾がゆがんでいる。

6-6 Misshapen digit 指趾形態異常 (Code No.: 10085, MP No.: 0002110, HP No.: 0001171)

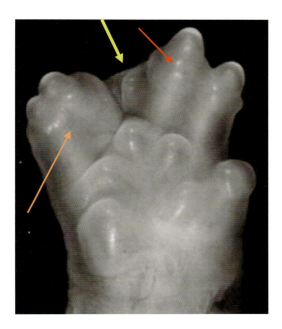

Species	Rat, Wistar
Memo	Misshapen digits of the fore-paw: Clinodactyly (10083, red arrow) and Syndactyly (10091, orange arrow) are observed. A web-like structure is observed between the 3rd and 4th digits (yellow arrow).
	形態異常指：第3指と第4指の間（黄色矢印）が空き、水かき様になっている（黄矢印）。斜指（10083、赤矢印）や合指（10091、オレンジ矢印）も伴う。

6-7　Pendulous digit　浮遊指　(Code No.: New)

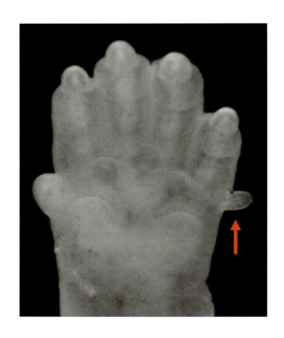

Species	Mouse, ICR
Memo	Pendulous digit of the fore-paw: Post-axial
	浮遊指：軸後性である。

6-7 Continued

Species	Rat, Wistar
Memo	Pendulous digit: Pendulous digit attach by a thread of tissue.
	浮遊指:索状組織でつながった有茎性の指趾である。

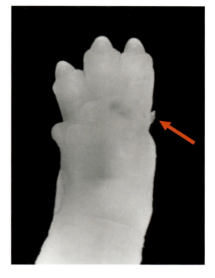
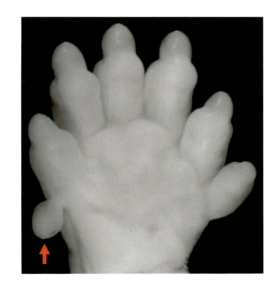
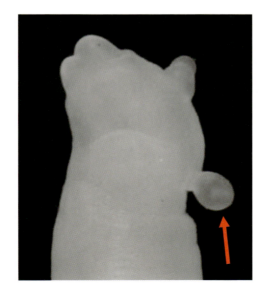
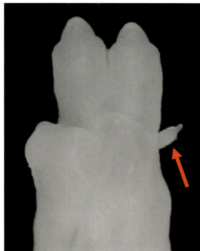

6-8 Small digit, Brachydactyly, Microdactyly 短指趾 (Code No.: 10079, MP No.: 0002544, HP No.: 0011927)

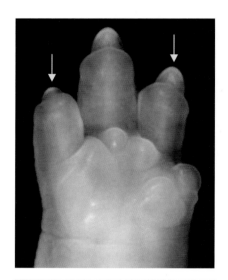

Species	Rat, Wistar
Memo	Brachydactyly or Microdactyly: Brachydactyly (arrow) with axial Oligodactyly (few digit).
	短指（矢印）：中軸性欠指（10080）も伴う。

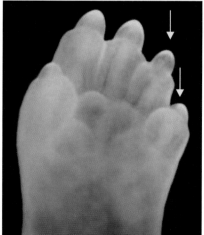

Species	Rat, Wistar
Memo	Brachydactyly, Microdactyly or Short digit: Shortening of the 4th and 5th digits of the hind-paw
	短趾、小趾：第4及び5趾が短い。

6-9 Supernumerary digit, Polydactyly 多指趾 (Code No.: 10088, MP No.: 0000562, HP No.: 0010442)

Species	Rat, Wistar
Memo	Polydactyly of the hind-paw: Pre-axial Polydactyly with Dactylomegaly (10081) of the hind-paw (arrows).
	多趾：軸前性、軸前性巨大趾（10081）を伴う。

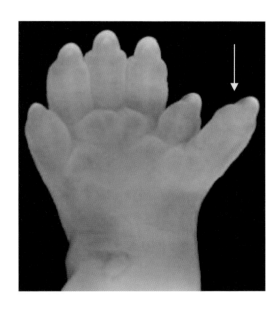 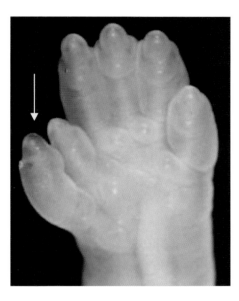

6-9 Continued

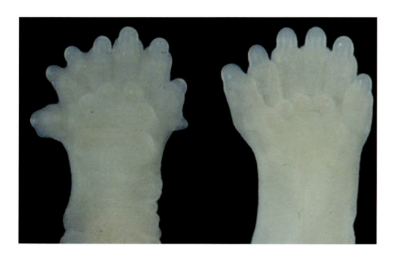

Species	Mouse, PDN
Memo	Left: Preaxial Polydactyly of fore-paw
	Right: Preaxial Polydactyly of hind-paw
	左：前肢軸前性多指
	右：後肢軸前性多趾

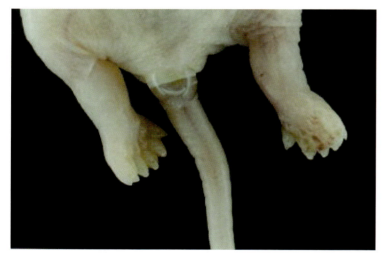

Species	Rat
Memo	Polydactyly of the hind-paw
	多趾

6-10　Absent claw　爪欠損　(Code No.: 10076, MP No.: 0008494, HP No.: 0001817)

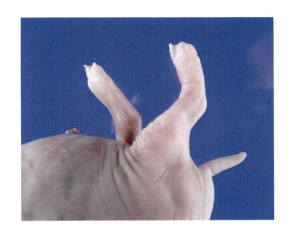

Species	Rabbit
Memo	Absent claw: The 3rd and 4th claws are absent.
	爪欠損：第3、4趾の爪欠損

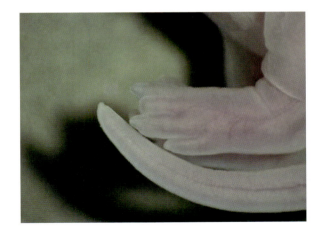

Species	Rat
Memo	Absent claw: The 3rd claw is absent.
	爪欠損：第3趾の爪が欠損している。

6-10 Continued

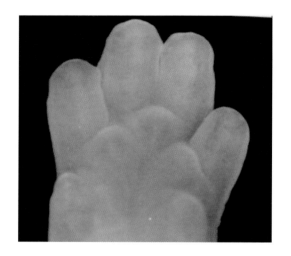

Species	Rat, Wistar
Memo	Absent claw of the fore-paw
	爪欠損：前肢

Species	Rat, Wistar
Memo	Absent claw of the hind-paw
	爪欠損：後肢

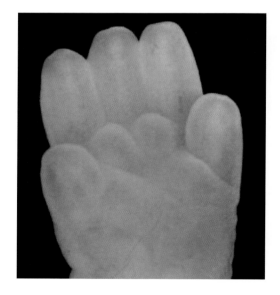

6-11 Small claw 爪小型化 (Code No.: 10089, MP No.: 0012399, HP No.: 0001804)

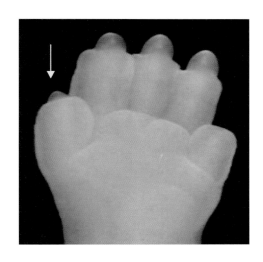

Species	Rat, Wistar
Note	Small claw with Absent claw (10076)
	爪小型化：爪欠損（10076）も伴う。

6-12 Malrotated paw 異常回転手足 (Code No.:10084)

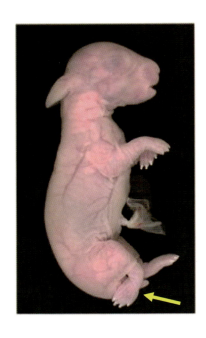

Species	Rabbit
Memo	Malrotated paw: Hind-paw turns laterally (arrow).
	異常回転足：外反足とも言う。足首から外側に向いている。

6-13　**Hyperflexion of paw**　過屈曲手　(Code No.: 10087)

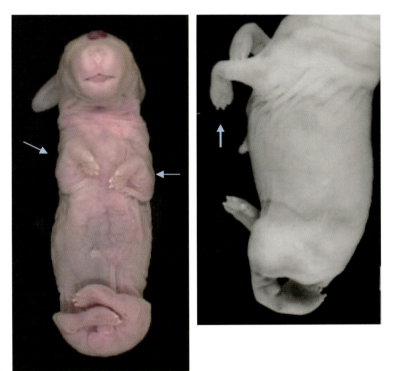

Species	Rabbit
Memo	Hyperflexion of the paw (fore-paw) or flexed paw with Malrotated hindlimb (both fetuses, 10072) and Meningo-encephalocele (left fetus, 10017)
	過屈曲手（前肢）：異常回転肢（後肢、10072）を伴う。左胎児は髄膜脳瘤（10017）も伴う。

6-13 Continued

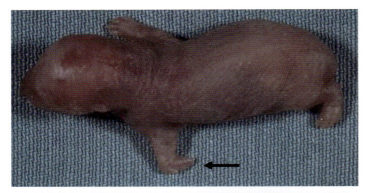

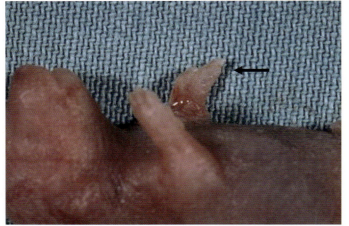

Species	Rat
Memo	Flexed paw with Oligodactyly (10080)
	前肢過屈手：欠指（10080）を伴う。

Photographs of External Anomalies

7. Tail

The tail is an animal-specific organ because it is a rudiment in human. External tail anomalies are divided into 4 categories: alterations in length, thickness, distal morphology and overall shape.

1. Alteration in length

1.1 Short tail or Brachyury (Code No. 10103): The tail is short.

1.2 Absent tail or Acaudate (Code No. 10093): The tail is absent or rudimentary.

1.3 Long tail (Code No. New): The tail is long.

2. Alteration in thickness

2.1 Blunt-tipped tail (Code No. 10095): The tip of the tail is rounded or flat, but not tapered.

2.2 Narrow tail or Constricted tail (Code No. 10102): The tail is constricted.

2.3 Thread-like tail (Code no. 10104): The tail is filamentous.

If abnormal parts of the tail fall off during the fetal period, Narrow tail and Thread-like tail cannot be identified and may be mistaken as Short tail or Absent tail.

3. Change in distal morphology

3.1 Bent tail (Code No. 10094): The tail is generally shaped like an angle.

3.2 Curled tail (Code No. 10096): The tail is curved into nearly a full circle, or coiled.

3.3 Hooked tail (Code No. 10099): The tail is bent or curved approximately 180 degree.

3.4 Kinked tail (Code No. 10100): The tail is generally curved twisting spirally.

4. Change in shape

4.1 Double-tipped tail, Bifurcated tail, or Duplicated tail (Code No. 10097): The tail is divided or split.

4.2 Fleshy tab of the tail or Small tag of the tail (Code No. 10098): The tail has small tag at the tip.

4.3 Malpositioned tail (Code No. 10101): The position of the tail is abnormal.

4.4 Discolored tail (Code No. New): Generalized or localized discoloration of the tail.

4.5 Misshapened tail (Code No. New): Abnormal shape except for above-mentioned anomalies.

尾は、ヒトにおいては外表として痕跡的であり、動物特有の組織と言える。尾の外表に認められる異常としては、長さ、太さ、走行、形の異常に大きく分けられる。

長さの異常は、短尾（尾が短い、Short tail、Code No. 10103）、無尾（尾がないあるいは痕跡状、Absent tail or Acaudate、Code No. 10093）及び長い尾（Long tail、Code No. New）である。

太さの異常としては、鈍端尾（尾先端が鈍、Blunt-tipped tail、Code No. 10095）、狭窄尾（尾が部分的に狭窄、Narrow tail、Code No. 10102）及び糸状尾（尾全体が細い、Thread-like tail、Code No. 10104）などがある。しかし、胎児期に異常な部分が脱落すれば、それぞれ、狭窄尾は短尾、糸状尾は無尾と区分できない場合もある。

走行の異常としては、屈曲尾（明らかに折れ曲がっている、Bent tail、Code No. 10094）、巻尾（ほぼ一巻している、あるいはコイル状になっている、Curled tail、Code No. 10096）、カギ状尾（180度折れ曲がっているか、弯曲している。Hooked tail、Code No. 10099）及び曲尾（尾の軸がネジの様にひねりながら全体として弯曲している。Kinked tail、Code No. 10100）などがある。これら走行の異常については、観察時に尾を一旦伸ばし、特徴的な変化であることを確認すべきである。また、巻尾と曲尾については良く似通っており、尾の血管などにより「ねじれ」を確認する。

形の異常としては、二又尾（あるいは分岐尾や重複尾、尾の基部あるいは中間部から分岐している。Bifurcated tail, Double-tipped tail, or Duplicated tail etc.、Code No. 10097）、尾肉様付属物（尾の先端に肉片あるいは皮膚の様な付属物がある。Fleshy tab of the tail or Small tag of the tail、Code No. 10098）尾位置異常（尾が通常外の場所に発生、Malpositioned tail、Code No. 10101）尾形態異常（上記のいずれにも該当しない形態異常、Misshapen tail、Code No. New）あるいは変色尾（尾の全体あるいは部分的な変色、Discolored tail、Code No. New）などがある。

なお、上記分類の中には骨格の異常が予測される変化も含まれるため、異常の本態を確認する必要がある場合は骨格検査が望ましい。仙尾椎の異常の写真を参考にされたい。

7-1   Absent tail, Anury, Acaudia   無尾   (Code No.: 10093, MP No.: 0003456)

Species	Rat
Memo	Acaudia, absent tail: This anomaly may include rudimentary tail.
	無尾：痕跡状のものも含めてもよい。

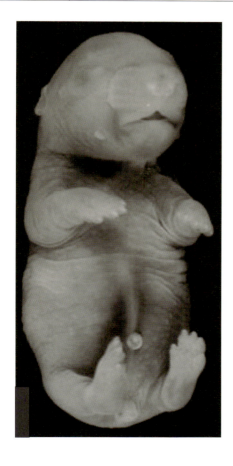
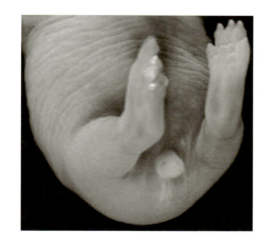
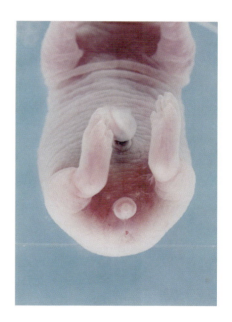

7-1 Continued

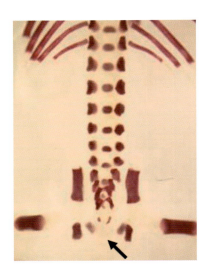

Species	Rat (Skeletal specimen)
Memo	Skeletal specimen of Anury: Fused sacral vertebral arches (10726) and Absent caudal vertebrae (10769) are observed.
	尾欠損の骨格例：仙椎弓の癒合（10726）と尾椎の欠損（10769）がみられる。

7-2　Bent tail　屈曲尾　(Code No.: 10094, MP No.: 0000585)

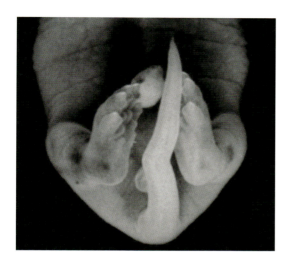

Species	Rat, Jcl:Wistar
Memo	Bent tail: Shaped like an angle. This observation should be distinguished from Curled (10096), Hooked (10099), or Kinked (10100) tail.
	尾屈曲：折れ曲がっている。典型的な写真 巻尾（10096）、カギ状尾（10099）、曲尾（10100）との区分けに注意。

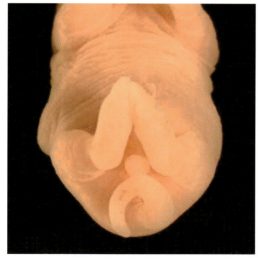

Species	Rat, Crl:CD(SD)
Memo	Bent tail: Shaped like an angle. This observation should be distinguished from Curled (10096), Hooked (10099), or Kinked (10100) tail.
	尾屈曲：折れ曲がっている。 巻尾（Curled tail, 10096）にも似ているが、不自然な屈曲部がみられる。 巻尾（10096）、カギ状尾（10099）、曲尾（10100）との区分けに注意。

7-2 Continued

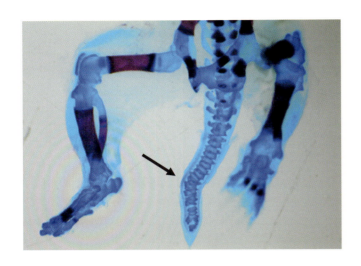

Species	Rat (Skeletal specimen)
Memo	Double-stained skeletal specimen of Bent tail: Fused (10763) and Misshapen (10767) caudal vertebral bodies at the bent point and the tip of the tail are observed.
	尾屈曲の骨格例（二重染色標本）：屈曲がみられる部分及び先端の尾椎体に癒合（10763）及び形態異常（10767）がみられる。

7-3　Bifurcated tail　二又尾　(Code No.: 10097, MP No.: 0013175)

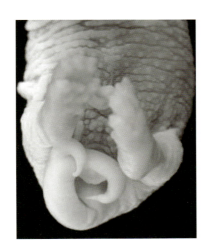

Species	Rat
Memo	Bifurcated tail, Double-tipped tail, Branched tail: Tail is divided or split.
	二又尾、分岐尾、フォーク状尾などと呼ばれる。分岐した尾がみられる。典型的な写真

Species	Rat
Memo	Bifurcated tail or Duplicated tail with Exencephaly: This fetus is considered to be Conjoined twins (see 1-2).
	二又尾、外脳を伴う。二重体の一種と考えられる（1-2 二重体参照）。

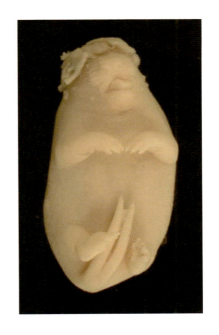

7-3 Continued

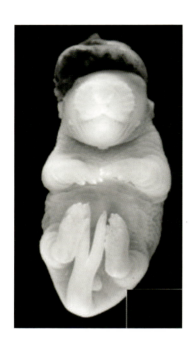

Species	Rat
Memo	Bifurcated tail with Exencephaly (10013): This fetus is considered to be Conjoined twins (see 1-2).
	二又尾、外脳（10013）を伴う。本例は骨格検査で脊柱管二重が認められている（1-2 二重体参照）。

Species	Rat
Memo	Bifurcated tail: The tip of the tail divides.
	二又尾：尾先端が二又になっている。

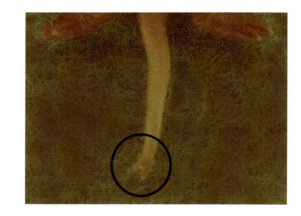

7-4 Curled tail 巻いた尾 (Code No.: 10096, MP No.: 0003051)

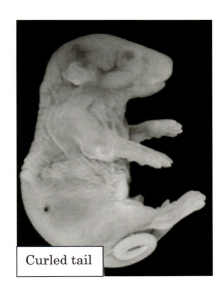

Species	Mouse
Memo	Curled tail: Tail is curved into a full circle.
	巻尾：尾が一巻している。

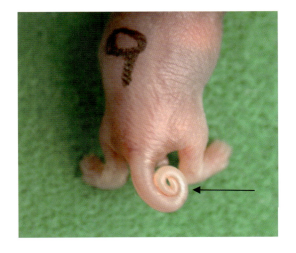

Species	Rat
Memo	Curled tail: Tail is curved into a full circle. It is confirmed that the shape of the tail vein is not spiral.
	巻尾：尾が一巻している。尾の血管に「ひねり」のないことが確認できる。

7-5 Fleshy tab tail　尾肉様付属物　(Code No.: 10098, MP No.: 0013177)

Species	Rat, Wistar
Memo	Fleshy tab tail: Small tag of the tissue at the tip of the tail. In this fetus, fleshy tab has hematoma.
	尾付属物：この写真は先端にtagがあり、この個体では先端部分が血腫になっている。

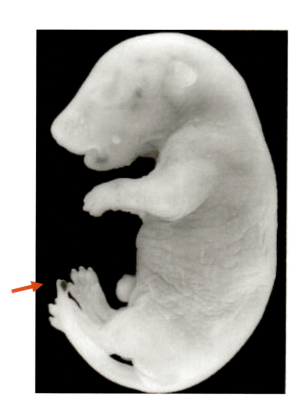

7-6　Hooked tail　カギ状尾　(Code No.: 10099, MP No.: 0002111)

Species	Rat
Memo	Hooked tail: Approximately 180 degree bend or curve of the tail.
	カギ状尾：尾が180°折れ曲がっているか／弯曲している。

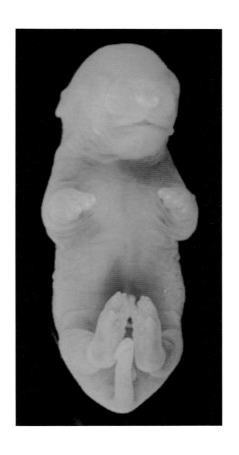
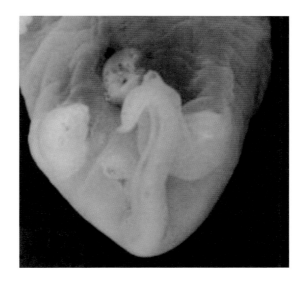

7-7 Kinked tail 曲尾   (Code No.: 10100, MP No.: 0003051)

Species	Rat
Memo	Kinked tail: It is difficult to differentiate between Kinked tail and Curled tail. This specimen with a Kinked tail shows a curled tail with a twisted axis of the tail. Note the direction of the tail blood vessel.
	曲尾（Kinked tail）：巻尾との判断が難しいが、本所見は尾の軸がネジの様にひねりながら全体として弯曲している。尾の動静脈の走行で確認するとよい。巻尾は「ひねり」がない。

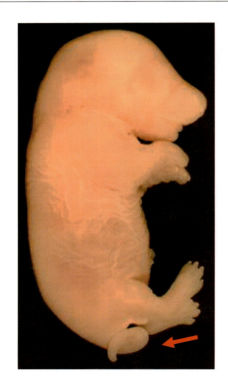

7-8 Misshapen tail 尾形態異常 (Code No.: New, MP No.: 0002111)

Species	Rat
Memo	Misshapen tail with duplicated penis: This fetus has duplicated tail; One tail is normal, and another tail is misshapen.
	尾形態異常：二重体の一種であり、尾と外部生殖器が重複して存在し、重複した一本の尾に形態異常が認められる。

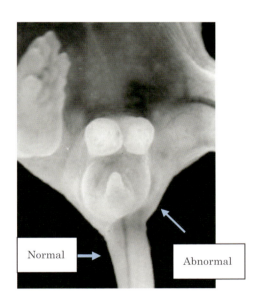

7-9 Narrow tail, Constricted tail 狭窄尾 (Code No.: 10102, MP No.: 0000589)

Species	Rat
Memo	Narrow tail, Constricted tail: All or a part of the tail is constricted (arrow). Should specify whether it is entire length or localized. 狭窄尾：尾の一部が狭窄している。基部、中間部、先端付近など位置は個体により異なるため、全体か特定の部位かを記載した方がよいかも知れない。

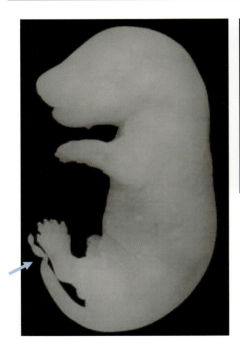
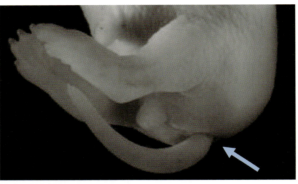
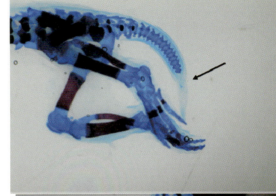
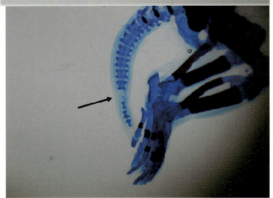

Right photographs

Skeletal specimens of Narrow tail: Absent caudal vertebrae (10769) is observed.

狭窄尾の骨格標本：尾椎の欠損（10769）が認められる。

7-10 Short tail, Brachyury 短尾 (Code No.: 10103, MP No.: 0000592)

Species	Rat
Memo	Shorter than normal length (Photos 1, 2 and 3): In rats and mice, if the tip of the tail does not reach or extend beyond the level of the point of attachment of the umbilicus, the tail will be judged to be "Short tail" (Photos 1 and 2). Specimen in Photo 3 may be considered to be "Anury (10093)".
	短尾：正常に比べ短い尾。ラット、マウスの場合、臍の位置より短いものを短尾と判断する。写真３の場合、無尾（10093）でもよいかも知れない。

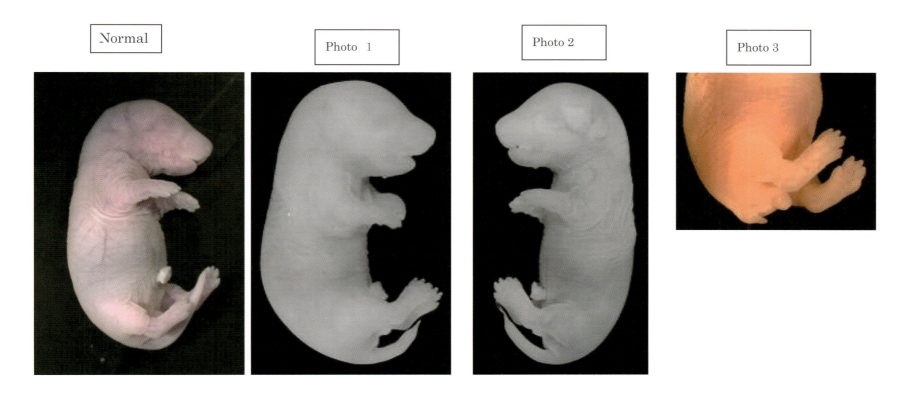

7-10 Continued

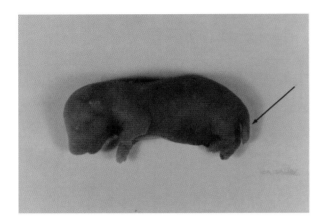

Species	Rat
Memo	Brachyury or Short tail
	短尾：尾が短い。

7-11 Thread-like tail 索状尾 (Code No.: 10104, MP No.: 0002632)

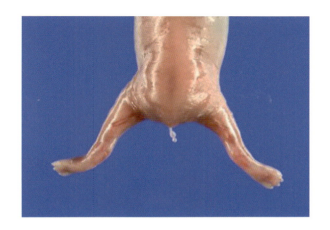

Species	Rabbit
Memo	Thread-like tail, Filamentous tail, Filiform tail: This may be "Anury (10093)" because this tail is rudimentary.
	索状尾、糸状尾：本例の場合は痕跡程度であり、無尾（10093）でもよいかも知れない。

Species	Rat
Memo	Thread-like tail, Filamentous tail, Filiform tail
	索状尾、糸状尾

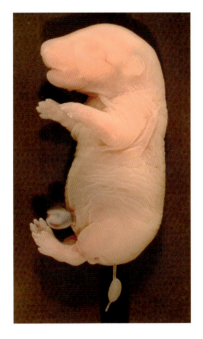
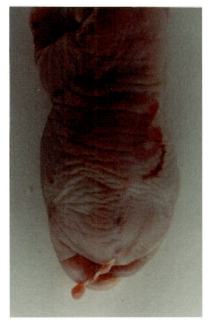

Photographs of External Anomalies

8. Trunk

8-1 Absent anus, Anal atresia 肛門欠損 (Code No.: 10105, MP No.: 0003130, HP No.: 0002023)

Species	Rat
Memo	Anal atresia, Aproctia, Imperforate anus or non-patent anus with Anury (10093): Absence or closure of the anal opening.
	鎖肛、肛門閉鎖、無肛門：肛門の欠損あるいは閉鎖、無尾（10093）を伴う。

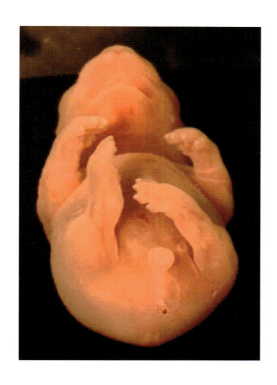
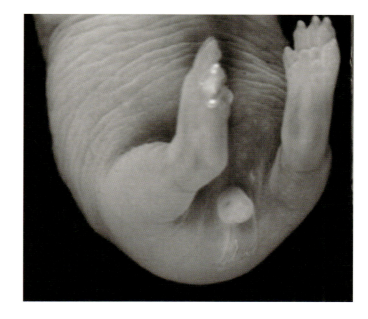

8-2 **Small anus** 肛門小型 (Code No.: 10118, MP No.: 0009052, HP No.: 0002025)

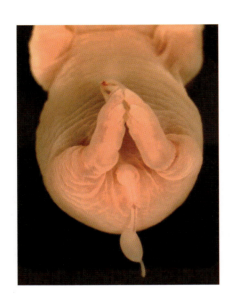

Species	Rat
Memo	Small anus with Thread-like tail (10104)
	肛門小型化、肛門狭窄：索状尾（10104）を伴う。

8-3 Externalized heart, Ectopia cordis 心臓逸所 (Code No.: 10108, MP No.: 0011660, HP No.: 0001683)

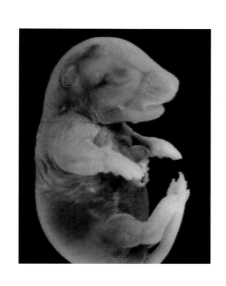 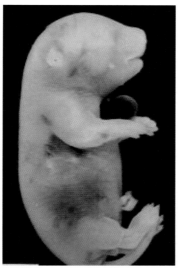

Species	Rat
Memo	Ectopia cordis: Heart displaced outside thoracic cavity.
	心臓逸所：胸腔外への心臓の逸脱、心臓のみ胸腔から突出している。

Right photograph
Skeletal specimen of fetus with Ectopia cordis: Split sternum or Sternoschisis (10619) is observed.
心臓逸所と思われる胎児の骨格標本：胸骨分離・胸骨裂（10619）が認められる。

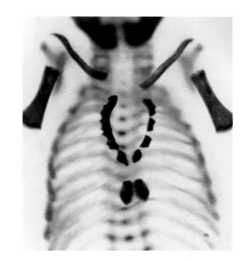

8-4　Gastroschisis　腹壁裂　(Code No.: 10109, MP No.: 0000757, HP No.: 0001543)

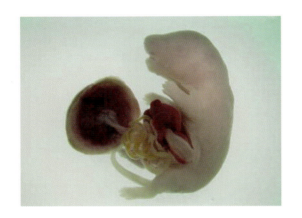

Species	Rat
Memo	Gastroschisis: Fissure of abdominal wall and protrusion of the viscera.
	腹壁裂：臍部以外の腹壁に裂が生じ、肝臓や腸管が露出している。露出した器官が膜性の嚢に覆われている場合もある。

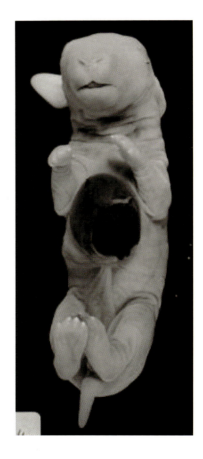

Species	Rabbit
Memo	Gastroschisis: Fissure of abdominal wall and protrusion of the liver; Need to distinguish Gastroschisis from Omphalocele (10115) and Umbilical hernia (10124).
	腹壁裂：臍部以外の腹壁に裂が生じ、肝臓が突出している。臍帯ヘルニア（10115、臍部の皮膚が欠損し、腸管が突出）や臍ヘルニア（10124、臍部の腹壁の欠損により腸管の突出：皮膚に覆われるか／臍輪から突出し、臍が隆起）と区別する。

8-5 Absent genital tubercle　生殖突起欠損　(Code No.: 10106)

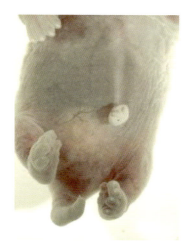

Species	Rat, Crl:SD
Memo	Absent genital tubercle with Short tail
	生殖突起欠損：短尾を伴っている。

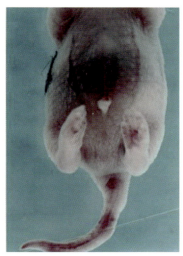 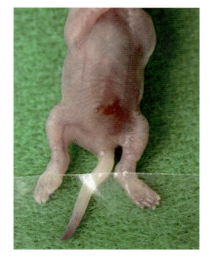

Species	Rat
Memo	Absent genital tubercle
	生殖突起欠損

8-6　Holorachischisis　完全脊椎裂　(Code No.: 10110, MP No.: 0008784)

Species	Mouse, Rat
Memo	Holorachischisis with Exencephaly (10013): Fissure of the entire spinal column
	完全脊椎裂：脊柱管全体に裂が生じている。外脳（10013）を伴っており、頭蓋脊柱破裂と総称される神経管閉鎖障害の一種。

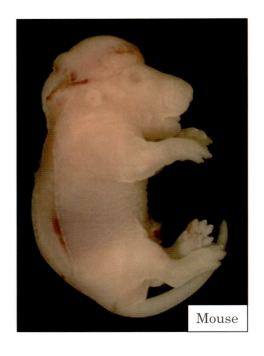
Mouse

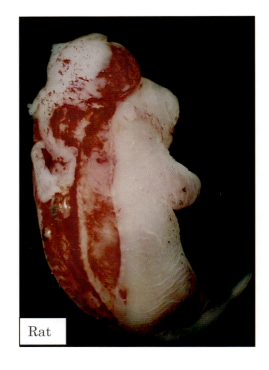
Rat

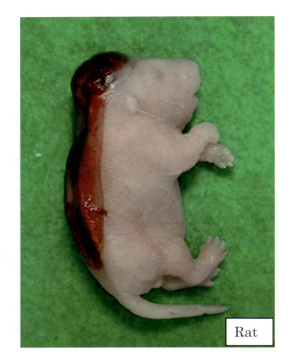
Rat

8-6 Continued

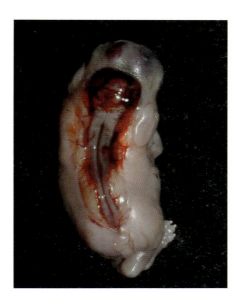

Species	Rabbit, Kbl:JW
Memo	Holorachischisis: Fissure of the entire spinal column
	完全脊椎裂：脊柱管全体に裂がみられる。

8-7 Hypospadias 尿道下裂 (Code No.: 10111, HP No.: 0000047)

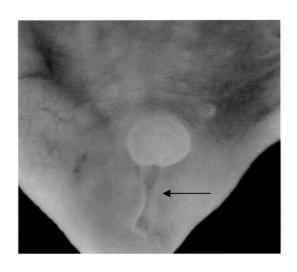

Species	Rat
Memo	Hypospadias: Fissure between genital tubercle and anus; It is difficult to observe the opening of the urethra in this fetus.
	尿道下裂：外生殖器と肛門の間に溝が見られる。胎児では尿道の開口を確認することは難しい。

8-8 Spina bifida 二分脊椎 (Code No.: 10120, MP No.: 0003054, HP No.: 0002414)

Species	Rabbit
Memo	Spina bifida at the lumbar region: A part of the spinal column is not close.
	二分脊椎（腰部）：脊柱管に部分的に裂が生じたものであり、通常、腰仙骨部にみられる。裂部が皮膚で覆われ、外表からは確認できず（潜在二分脊椎）、椎弓欠損等の骨格異常として認められることもある。"神経管閉鎖障害"の一種

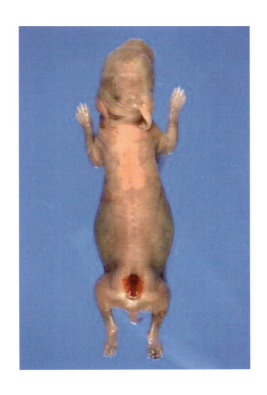
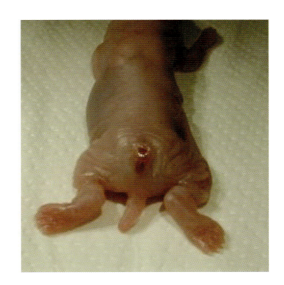

8-8 Continued

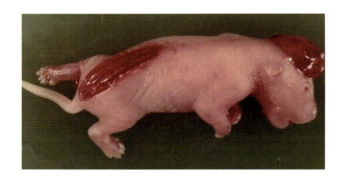

Species	Rat
Memo	Spinal bifida with Eyelid fissure (Open eyelid, 10034) and Exencephaly (10013)
	二分脊椎：眼瞼裂（10031）及び外脳（10037）を伴う。

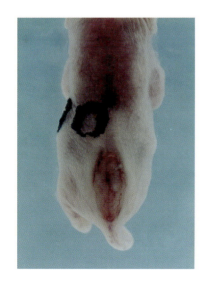

Species	Rat
Memo	Spina bifida at the lumbar region
	二分脊椎（腰部）

8-9 Thoracogastroschisis 胸腹壁裂 (Code No.: 10121, MP No.: 0000757, HP No.: 0100656)

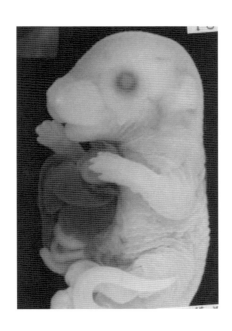

Species	Mouse, KK-A^y
Memo	Thoracogastroschisis: Fissure of thoracic and abdominal walls with the heart, liver, intestines etc. exposed ventrally.
	胸腹壁裂：胸腹壁の裂により、心臓、肝臓、腸管などが突出している。

8-9 Continued

Species	Rabbit
Memo	Thoracogastroschisis: Fissure of thoracic and abdominal walls
	胸腹壁裂：胸腹壁の裂により、胸腹部器官が突出している。

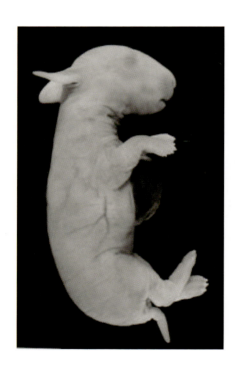
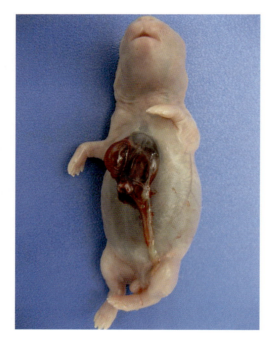

Right photograph
Skeletal specimen of fetus with Thoracogastroschisis: Split sternum or Sternoschisis (10619) is observed.
胸腹壁裂の骨格標本：胸骨分離（10619）が認められる。

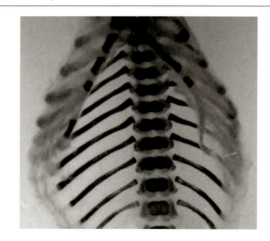

8-10 Small trunk, Short trunk 　短躯　 (Code No.: 10117, MP No.: 0001258, HP No.: 0003521)

Species	Rat
Memo	Short trunk with Micromelia of the hindlimb (10073, both specimens) and Anury (10093, left specimen)
	短躯：後肢小肢（10073、両図）及び無尾（10093、左図）を伴う。

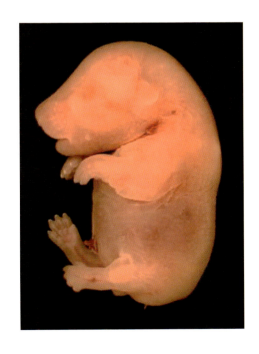
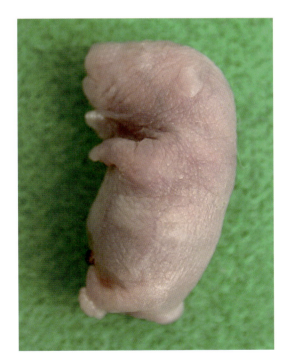

8-10 Continued

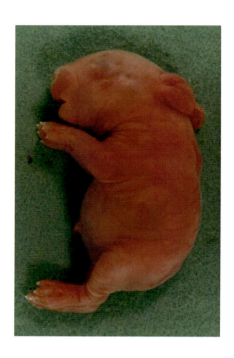

Species	Rabbit
Memo	Short trunk with and Anury (10093)
	短躯：無尾（10093）を伴う。

8-11　Omphalocele　臍帯ヘルニア　(Code No.: 10115, MP No.: 0003052, HP No.: 0001539)

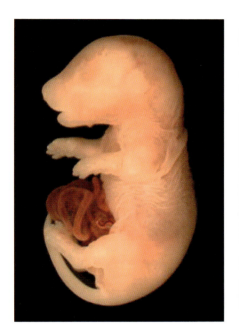 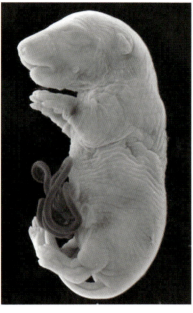

Species	Rat
Memo	Omphalocele: A defect in the abdominal wall at the umbilicus and protrusion of the intestines; Need to distinguish Omphalocele from Gastroschisis (10109) and Umbilical hernia (10124).
	臍帯ヘルニア：臍部の皮膚（腹壁）が欠損し、腸管などが突出している。薄い膜に覆われている場合もある。腹壁裂（10109、腹壁の裂により肝臓や腸管が突出）と臍ヘルニア（10124、臍部の腹壁の欠損による腸管の突出、皮膚に覆われるか／臍が隆起）と区分する。

8-12　Umbilical hernia　臍ヘルニア　(Code No.: 10124, MP No.: 0010146, HP No.: 0001537)

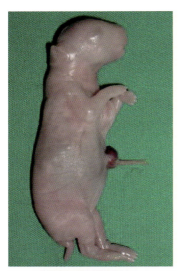

Species	Rabbit, Kbl:JW
Memo	Umbilical hernia: A defect in the abdominal wall at the umbilicus. This anomaly is covered by a thin, translucent sac composed of peritoneum and amnion; Need to distinguish this from Omphalocele (10115) and Gastroschisis (10109).
	臍ヘルニア：臍部の腹壁の欠損により腸管の突出：皮膚に覆われるか／臍輪から突出し、臍が隆起している。腹壁裂（10109、臍部以外の腹壁に裂が生じ、肝臓が突出している）や臍帯ヘルニア（10115、臍部の皮膚が欠損し、腸管が突出）と区別する。

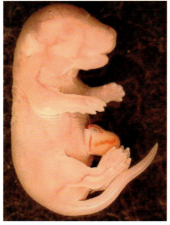

Species	Mouse
Memo	Umbilical hernia : A defect in the abdominal wall at the umbilicus. This anomaly is covered by a thin, translucent sac composed of peritoneum and amnion; Need to distinguish this from Omphalocele (10115) and Gastroschisis (10109).
	臍ヘルニア：臍部の腹壁の欠損により腸管の突出：皮膚に覆われるか／臍輪から突出し、臍が隆起している。腹壁裂（10109、腹壁に裂が生じ、肝臓が突出している）や臍帯ヘルニア（10115、臍部の皮膚が欠損し、腸管が突出）と区別する。

Atlas of Developmental Anomalies in Experimental Animals
実験動物発生異常アトラス

External Anomalies
外表異常

2015 年 3 月 10 日　第 1 刷発行

編集　日本先天異常学会用語委員会
Edited by Project of the Terminology Committee of the Japanese Teratology Society

発行　株式会社 薬事日報社　YAKUJI NIPPO, LTD.
　　　http://www.yakuji.co.jp
　　　本社　東京都千代田区神田和泉町 1
　　　電話　(03) 3862-2141
　　　支社　大阪市中央区道修町 2-1-10
　　　電話　(06) 6203-4191

印刷・製本　昭和情報プロセス株式会社

落丁本・乱丁本はお取り替えいたします。本書の無断複製を禁じます。